TOO YOUNG
TO GROW OLD

TAKE CONTROL OF YOUR HEALTH NOW!

ANNE-LISE MILLER

TOO YOUNG TO GROW OLD

First published in Great Britain by
Fisher King Publishing Ltd.

Fisher King Publishing Ltd
The Studio
Arthington Lane
Pool in Wharfedale
LS21 1JZ
England
www.fisherkingpublishing.co.uk

Project Manager: Francine Lawrence
Designer: Nicola Yuen
Cover Design: Nicola Yuen
Food Photography: Francine Lawrence

With additional assistance from:
Lorraine Jerram
Victoria Barrett
Vanessa Bird
Susi Hoyle

A CIP catalogue record of this book is available from the British Library
ISBN 978-1-910406-30-4

9293169

TOO YOUNG TO GROW OLD

ANNE-LISE MILLER

Foreword by

Dr Nick Read MA, MD, FRCP
Gastroenterologist, Physiologist, Nutritionist, Psychotherapist
Author of *Sick and Tired: Healing the Illnesses Doctors Cannot Cure*

FOREWORD

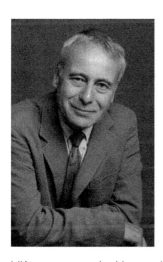

When I was a medical student in the 1960s the diseases we studied were the old ones: infections such as tuberculosis, smallpox, poliomyelitis, diphtheria. We don't see those now; vaccination, hygeine, and antibiotics have all but eradicated them. Heart attacks, cancer and stroke are now the major killers, but were they always there waiting to strike if people lived long enough – or is there something toxic about life in the 21st century?

As those major infections have faded from the developed Western world, doctors and their patients have become more sensitive to 'stress-related', 'lifestyle' and auto-immune diseases. GPs' surgeries and out-patient clinics throughout the UK are crammed with people with hay fever, asthma, coeliac disease, diabetes, irritable bowel syndrome, lupus, autistic spectrum disorder, depression, Crohn's Disease and a plethora of other allergic and immunological diseases, some of which were unknown 50 years ago.

Millions of people are racked by back pains, tormented by abdominal gripes, alarmed by ringing in their ears, tortured by headaches, exhausted by sleep deprivation, frustrated with constipation, debilitated with nausea and faintness, overwhelmed by the burden of obesity, terrified by shortness of breath or palpitations or just too sick and tired to cope. Such everyday illnesses may not kill them but they seriously compromise their comfort, mobility, pleasure of eating and social interaction. Too many people, it seems, are getting old before their time.

Disease occurs as a result of the interaction between us and our environment. The changes that have occurred in the way we live, the food we eat, the work we do, even the air we breathe and the water we drink can alter the expression not only of our human genome but also the far greater number of genes that encode for the metabolism of the myriad micro-organisms that live on us and inside us. Together these affect the sensitivity of our immune surveillance and our neuroendocrine control, resetting the function of our mind and body and releasing a new kind of malaise, for which traditional medicine, a pill for every ill, no longer applies.

In her book, *Too Young to Grow Old*, Anne-Lise Miller proposes that modern illnesses are the interaction of the changes induced in our bodily systems by our food, our activity, the stress we are under, our beliefs, the toxins we consume and

"40% of the British population now consider themselves to have a long term illness; 60% are overweight."

the medicines we take. Health, she asserts, is no longer the prerogative of health professionals. 'Health' services are not good at keeping people well. While they may claim to promote 'evidence-based' healthy solutions for individual systemic illness, 'we are all vulnerable to the influence of externally validated truths'.

The strength of this attractively presented oeuvre is its philosophical approach. Health and wellbeing, Ms Miller asserts, is our own personal responsibility, a matter of choice, an ongoing process of adapting our beliefs and behaviour to the changes that occur in our lives, realising our creativity and changing the outcome.

Too Young to Grow Old offers a smorgasbord of practical solutions. These include advice on sleep hygiene, exercise, stress management, healthy eating, the balance of work and life, creativity, nature and the environment and ways to facilitate the elimination of toxins that accumulate in our bodies as a result of the way we live. Treatment of lifestyle illnesses do not have to be about deprivation. We can discover pleasure and a sense of balance in a positive and healthy approach to eating, exercise, work and society.

This book is a *tour de force;* a rich blend of ancient wisdom and modern science. Take the time to read it thoughtfully. Explore the sections that resonate with you, take from those the ideas that seem to help, engage, realise less is often more, commit to meaningful change, but pace yourself, allow time to make it a habit, find your own way. Living longer need not be a gradual deterioration in function and wellbeing, it can be a celebration of wisdom and experience and the youthful vitality to enjoy them.

Dr Nick Read MA, MD, FRCP
Gastroenterologist, Physiologist, Nutritionist, Psychotherapist.
Author: *Sick and Tired: Healing the Illnesses Doctors Cannot Cure.*

ABOUT ME

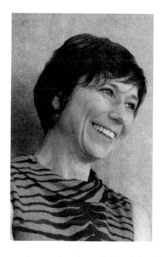

I was born in Paris 50 years ago at a time when French society had recovered from the ravages of war but before cultural fragmentation and the rise of feminism. French identity and values were based on socialism, equality and the comforting gift of philosophy shared among friends – usually enjoyed with the help of a good bottle of wine and delicious home cooked food.

I came to London to study contemporary dance when I was 19 and I discovered the British culture with its quirky individuality, feminist views and exotic multi-cultural society. It may seem odd now, but in 1983 the clash was spectacular. It challenged and irrevocably formed my identity. I discovered wholefoods and vegetarian restaurants; alongside white sliced bread, tasteless iceberg lettuces and fruit sold by the piece – unheard of in France at that time!

Dance turned out to be my therapy, but not my passion. Through it I realised the pitfalls of pursuing looks and ideals instead of health; and felt the pain of trying to conform to standards that were neither my own, nor physically possible. I smoked, drank a lot of coffee and my body ached most of the time. For a few years, I went on fighting the image I stared at daily in the huge mirrors of the dance studios until the day I decided that this was not for me and I set out on the journey towards my true vocation.

With dance I had developed an acute awareness of my body and the kinesiology of movement – or more precisely how proper alignment guarantees the minimum effort for the maximum impact. Muscles had to be coordinated and balanced to ensure optimum results I began to study physical therapies and discovered that I could physically tune into a client's muscles when I massaged them and receive a multitude of silent information. I would get to know the person through their tension and the response of their body to my touch. I could help and guide them, but I could not do it for them. Each person had to find their own path and their own realignment, but I had found my true vocation. In 1992, I undertook two-year training in Systematic Kinesiology with Brian Butler and gradually realised that the principles of self-adjustment and balance could also be applied to personality and life-style. I eventually developed my own way of working and supporting my clients to reclaim their health through better self-awareness, lifestyle choices, dietary adjustment – and regular detoxes.

In 1998 I opened a detox retreat in Scotland with my husband at a time when

"Too often what we gain in wisdom, we lose in vitality. I am convinced this does not have to be the case."

the concept had not yet been born. I became privy to the extraordinary healing potential of fasting and detoxing. People would transform before our eyes in a matter of days. The following 15 years I spent in Scotland were a great opportunity to experiment on my own health, and learn from the numerous guests who came to stay with us.

Today I can sincerely say that I feel healthier than I was at 20, my body is stronger and pain-free, my weight stable and my moods far more consistent. I have found strategies to control my weaknesses and feel more confident in my strength. The wisdom of self-knowledge is undoubtedly the product of time, but too often what we gain in wisdom we lose in vitality. I am convinced this does not have to be the case.

A few years ago I was diagnosed with a rare genetic disease which, I was told, would result in blindness akin to macular degeneration and was unavoidable with age. The signs were all there in my retina and two years ago my vision was affected by black spots and wavy lines. I was told that the condition was in my genes and that because of my age more deterioration was inevitable and I would have to accept it. Instead, despite my parents' concern I challenged the doctors' prognosis and faced my own fears. I increased my antioxidants, removed gluten from my diet and detoxed my liver – nothing too extreme – but six months later I was rewarded with straight lines and no black spots. I still remember the day I looked out of the window and it dawned on me that everything was clear and at last my vision was normal.

So many of the people I have accompanied along the way to health recovery have encouraged me to write about my experience and approach. It is to them, and the many more who continue to regularly consult me in London and take part on my week long detox retreats, that I dedicate this book.

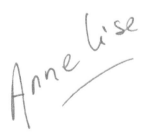

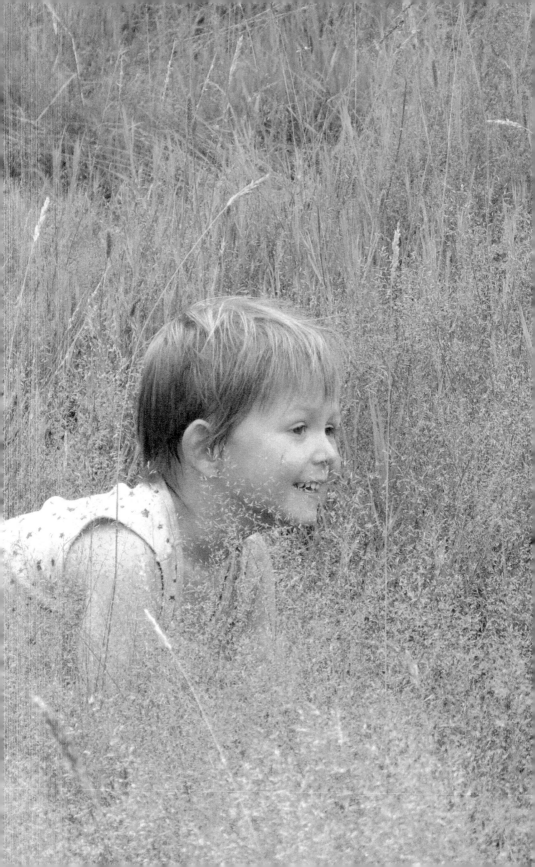

WHEN DO WE START TO GROW 'OLD'?

In our collective consciousness there is a solidly held belief that health wanes with age. I challenge that belief. While ageing is a natural biological process, health is the consequence of dynamic and multiple interactions between our unique biology, personality, lifestyle and environment. We can look after our health and sustain it – regardless of age. This book is not just another health manual or a 'get well quick' method, but a compendium of vital health facts, nutritional information and scientifically proven research that I have collected and put into practice during my 30 years of seeing and successfully treating hundreds of clients.

When do we stop growing up and start to grow old? At what point do we become conscious that our physical fitness and our appearance have evolved on a path all of their own? Which life event, which encounter suddenly jerks us to the realisation that something is happening to us and nothing will ever be the same? The realisation that we no longer have all the time in the world is never a happy moment. Yet, it is only by *embracing* the challenges that come with ageing that we can ensure that we remain fit and healthy, and able to enjoy a rich and fruitful life well into our 80s and 90s. In fact there are now more people in the world than ever before who reach 100 and are in good health. The number of centenarians is doubling every ten years in the western world. Progress in psychology, physiology, nutrition and medicine makes it a very likely prospect that we will all live to a greater age than our parents, so we had better start preparing for it.

Our current western culture mistakenly venerates youth, which is actually unattainable because it is in constant evolution. Good health, on the other hand, is specific to the individual whatever their age, and therefore possible to aim for. Health is not relative to external perception, such as matching an image in a magazine, but is defined by how we *feel*...or so it should be!

Connecting with how we feel physically, mentally and emotionally is the paradigm shift required to positively embrace health and anti-ageing. By integrating our physical and mental perceptions we connect with our ability to adapt, thrive and be healthy throughout all our life. We can radiate the kind of beauty which comes from within and is timeless. The fact that health doesn't just feel good but also looks good is evidence of its relevance in a programme designed to control ageing. However, too often appearance is the aim rather than the consequence. 'Diets' are sold on the basis that they will help us slim and a multitude of face creams claim to make wrinkles disappear, with little reference to what is happening internally. Healthy weight and beautiful skin are external symptoms of health and go hand in hand with healthy arteries, emotional wellbeing, good digestion – and many other factors.

The symptoms of good health are rarely defined. Common belief tells us that 'health' is the opposite of disease; therefore if you aren't ill then you must be healthy. If a doctor can't find a disease to explain the absence of health then the cause must be mental (or psychosomatic!). An integrated approach does not treat disease but *aims to improve health*. This is an important foundation in our self-perception and one that fully restores the power we all have to influence our wellbeing and our ageing experience.

This book combines recent research-based evidence in nutrition and bio-chemistry with developments in psychology. While the former demonstrates the importance of diet and nutrients on a wide range of functions from immune to cardiovascular, the latter improves our understanding of what exactly makes us happy and how we have been misled by valuing other aspects of our life. This is an essential part of my message because in our profit-based world, economics rather than health is designed to drive our behaviour. In the eyes of marketing specialists, health is just another commodity; something to aspire to and fail, so we have to buy more goods to fix the problem.

Contrary to popular belief, health isn't a gift that we have received through good fortune and over which we have little control. Nor is it a simple measurement of good behaviour. It is far more complex, and results from the connection between our personal interpretation of health and the acceptance of what and who we are. Our experience of health is the result of a myriad of choices and interactions between our physiology, our psychology and our environment. To best support good health, we need a reliable source of valid information and we need to be more conscious of what motivates us. However, the aim isn't to lead a perfect and regimented lifestyle, but to become more accepting of who we are and learn what suits and supports us.

The more we understand that connection between our beliefs, our perception and our choices, the healthier our experience of life will feel.

Your body is a complex and wonderful thing that influences and is influenced by your mind; they cannot be separated and the result makes you unique. This holistic approach is proven on a daily basis by anthropologists, biologists and bio-chemists who understand that no living organism, system or molecule exists on its own and that an action at any level will affect the rest of the system.

With ageing we acquire knowledge and experience. Providing we are aware we may even sense if something feels right or not and develop "inner wisdom" about what suits us as a result. However, too often circumstances and old habits conspire against that inner knowing, leading us to make choices with disastrous consequences such as chronic disease, obesity and premature ageing.

Currently obesity is the biggest health issue threatening global populations. It was recently estimated that its impact across the world has taken over that of hunger[1]. Excess of the wrong food now kills three times as many as lack of food. This sad fact is compounded by the absolute failure of policies applied across the western world for the last 40 years on the populations' weight management. Since the 1970s governments, medics and publicists have been telling us that we are getting fat because we consume too many calories, therefore we must cut down on the food that contains more than twice as much as any other foods: FAT. This assertion marked the advent of a global health disaster. In theory, each isolated piece of information that continues to be perpetuated to this day through the media and health services is true: too many calories do lead to excess weight and obesity; fat does contain a lot of calories; and fructose does not raise blood sugar (and therefore could be looked at as an alternative to sugar for diabetics); BUT put together those recommendations have not produced the anticipated results because food is not just about calories. Diabetes is not just about raised blood sugar – the combined effect of antibiotics and artificial substances like sweeteners is so detrimental to overall physiology that they do more harm than the supposed calories they are saving us from.

It is time for a different approach and for each one of us to become more discerning.

If you believe that the nutritional and lifestyle choices you make influence your health and wellbeing, and that your mental attitude dramatically influences your ability to thrive in a world that is challenging to your health, then read on!

---

1 http://www.telegraph.co.uk/health/healthnews/9742960/Obesity-killing-three-times-as-many-as-malnutrition.html

Too Young to Grow Old

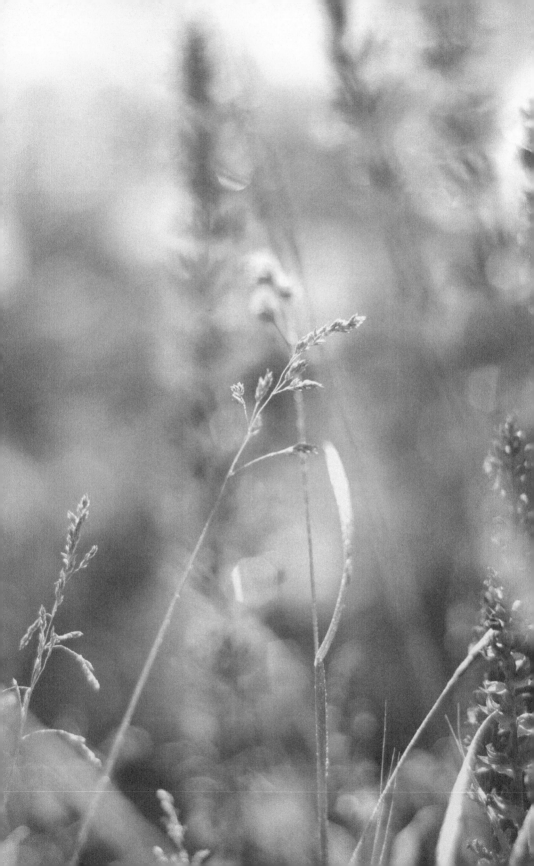

PART ONE:
TAKE CONTROL!

*"You are never too old to set another goal
or to dream a new dream."*

C. S. LEWIS

WHAT IS 'GOOD HEALTH' ANYWAY?

Every one of my patients has taught me something and helped develop my approach to health and longevity. However, some of the more significant realisations that shaped the philosophy behind my approach resulted from challenging the perceived wisdom habitually associated with health and healing.

HEALTH IS A FLEXIBLE CONCEPT

The World Health Organisation tells us "health is a state of complete physical, mental and social wellbeing and not merely the absence of disease or infirmity". Health is also a personal interpretation and an individual experience. If I ask 20 people to give me their symptoms of good health we'll probably agree on most of them, but after years of listening, advising and observing my clients I have concluded that health itself lies in our ability to connect personal perception, belief and behaviour with the choices we make daily. Health can be measured by the coherence of our choices with our Self as much as by the experience we have of it. The most significant step we can take towards maintaining our health is to become aware of those choices, what drives them and if they are actually in step with our beliefs and perceptions. As we will see in this book this is far from obvious and is not limited to food and exercise choices.

Most people, practitioners included, believe that for every symptom there must be a remedy and the expertise lies in identifying the correct one. While at a very simplistic level this logic works (we can sometimes cure a headache with Paracetamol), when we look more closely this cannot be true because symptoms of health and symptoms of disease result from complex and individual sets of interactions.

Managing our health is less about who has the right answer and more about which answer suits us best. Only when we examine what makes us who we are, can we know and decide *our* needs; until we reach that understanding of ourselves, we tend to just blindly follow whoever is the most persuasive with their argument or who promises to make it all ok for us.

The realisation that managing our health is our own responsibility is a challenging thought. It breaks the illusion that our medical health service will be there to look after us in our times of need or that medical authority is reassuringly godlike and capable of "fixing" us. However personal responsibility carries profound hope.

It restores the extraordinary power we all have to directly influence our health. This doesn't mean that medical health practitioners don't have anything to offer, far from it. It simply means that by committing to our health we engage the whole of our Self in that process and optimise the result.

A HEALTHY BALANCED DIET DOESN'T EXIST

In my practice if I ask details about someone's diet their response will usually be "I have a healthy diet but …". What follows varies; it could be "I eat too late at night or I snack or I eat too much chocolate".

What interests me most in their response is what comes before the "but". What is a healthy diet? Healthy for what? Who says it's healthy? How do they know?

Most people define a healthy diet in relation to what is published by health agencies and governments. We are advised to eat low fat foods, five to seven fruits and vegetables per day and be mindful of our calorie intake because otherwise we will get fat and fat is bad news! Simple…

This type of message is so general that it is absurd. It does not address the question of individual requirements for essential nutrients, the fact that diet must be applied to lifestyle (an office worker does not have the same requirements as those of an athlete) and that the nutritional content of a particular food varies considerably depending on cooking, growing method and freshness. The food industry is always ready to exploit those messages to its advantage, regardless of the true benefits to our health, and yet the majority of people, and health workers alike, believe in the myth of the 'healthy diet'.

If it is true that a bad diet can easily be defined, the reverse is impossible. There is no 'good diet', there is only the diet, which is adapted to the individual. This has to take into consideration taste, culture, lifestyle, activity and emotional needs, as well as pathology. For example, the generally agreed virtues of a diet rich in fresh vegetables is put into question when bowel flora is severely disturbed, that is when fibre can become harmful and consequently fibre-rich vegetables need to be controlled. There is no point in adopting any kind of diet without first ensuring that it suits us as individuals and is adapted to our lifestyle. A young active person doesn't have the same needs as an older more sedentary grandparent.

HEALING ONLY EVER COMES FROM WITHIN

Healing is a functional process and the consequence of the interactive and continuously adjusting equilibrium maintained by our various physiological systems. It can be encouraged, supported and influenced by a variety of "remedies" but it is only the result of the interactions between the interventions (therapy, medication, etc) and our body. No healing takes place as a direct result of medication even if this is what we observe. For instance, a life threatening infection can clear after a course of antibiotics and lead us to think that the antibiotics are responsible for this small miracle. In actual fact the miracle is coming from our immune system which was able to recover with the assistance of the antibiotic. Yet it is entirely possible that the same antibiotic could interact in the opposite way and send us into anaphylactic shock. The same medication can have a very different result. It is not the medication but the interactions with our physiology, psychology and circumstances.

The usual expectation when someone consults me is to heal. Many practitioners call themselves healers and complementary health is sometimes referred to as the healing art. While healing implies reaching a static state of being (I am now healed), health is an on-going process of adaptation and a truer representation of our physiology.

'Healthy' is the result of our ability to adapt and constantly adjust to what we do, our environment and our mental state. Symptoms are useful measurements of progress but if restricted to a diagnosis can become a measurement of failure. Breast cancer, for instance, may refer to particular test results on breast tissues but how many other symptoms are parts of that experience? Those symptoms have probably developed over many years before the final diagnosis was made and already tell us where we can make changes even before we have to decide on cancer treatments.

Sometimes healing is just one of the possible outcomes from better health management. By concentrating on health rather than (medical) symptoms we can shift our focus away from the possibility of failure. To harness our health potential cannot be a failure while "not healing" can. Sickness and health need not be opposite but both expressions of the complex interactions that govern our health.

WELLBEING IS ALSO A PHILOSOPHY

The therapeutic philosophy of my approach seeks to harmonise our choices and objectives. Most health problems, and especially premature ageing, are rooted in incongruences. Those can simply be between our physiology and what we choose to eat. For instance we know that we really don't need to eat that dessert but choose to ignore the voice of reason. More subtly, it can be between what we believe to be healthy and what we choose to do, such as avoiding the gym on the way home despite having recently joined. But the more insidious incoherencies come from the discrepancy between what we feel we should be and who we actually are. This is what happens when we feel trapped and

A HARD PILL TO
SWALLOW!

14,000

is the estimated average number of prescribed tablets swallowed by each person in Britain in their lifetime. This does not include pills we might buy over the counter, which would total about

40,000 PILLS EACH

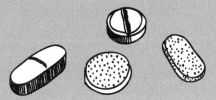

http://www.theguardian.com/commentisfree/2012/feb/17/pills-medicine-ian-jack

believe that we are a victim of circumstance. This belief renders us powerless and relentlessly chips away at the possibility of regaining control over our wellbeing.

OUR EMOTIONAL (STRESS) STATE DOESN'T DEFINE US BUT REFLECTS OUR HEALTH STATE

When I grew up tantrums were described as attention seeking and were reprimanded, while displays of affection were encouraged. This had the effect of making me believe that emotional reactions could be good and desirable, or bad and best avoided altogether. I didn't understand that the problem was the behaviour and not the emotion.

Emotions are simply what we feel. The physical sensation we have learned to register as sad, joyful, angry or affectionate is how we know that we are in that particular emotional state. A specific level of tension at the pit of the stomach, a mouth that feels dry, a throat that tightens ever so slightly, a set of facial muscles that arrange themselves in the corresponding manner are all so intimately linked to an emotional state that it is impossible to tell them apart or know where it starts or what precisely emotions are made of.

To deny our feelings is like disconnecting from the physical clues that inform us and feed into our consciousness, and the appraisal of situations and people we interact with. Those very same feelings also teach us if a choice is useful or harmful. They help us learn life's lessons, understand others better and connect with what is around us.

Recognising and welcoming my feelings (all of them) was a liberating moment for me. By acknowledging rather than denying them, I saw that feelings were not only transient but the product of a physiological state. Anyone who has felt irrational or angry because of hunger, stress or pre-menstrual tension knows the pitfalls of believing that emotions define us, yet most us forget just how much emotions are defined by our physical health and bio-chemical state.

To distinguish what we feel from what we are is also a fundamental step toward a more integrated understanding of health and self-empowerment. "I am depressed" (which is so often what people say to me) becomes: "I feel low/ heavy/confused/tearful/lacking in confidence, etc" and these are valuable clues to assess and measure where I am at this particular moment.

To see our emotions as representative of the relationships between our mental, physical and physiological state allows for a kinder and more hopeful perspective on ourselves. In this book I discuss simple practical measures and adjustments that can powerfully influence and modify emotional states.

HEALTH IS THE EXPRESSION OF AN IMPRESSION

A recent experiment in Finland on 701 subjects from different cultural backgrounds[1] demonstrated that similar emotions are perceived in similar physical ways, suggesting that feelings have a common physical reality regardless of cultural background. The researchers were able to develop a universal mapping system to visually represent emotions and their physically perceived sensations, which may partly explain how emotions, if experienced for long periods of time can specifically impact on health. This begs the question of what comes first: the belief that a particular emotional state is encoded in a set of physical responses, or if a particular sensation is synonymous with an emotion that we are used to naming – such as love or anger? What we can conclude is that beliefs and expectations are as much part of our emotions as is our physiology.

When it comes to ageing, the most damaging belief is that ageing means a gradual loss of wellbeing, an unavoidable string of unpleasant symptoms and a slow rejection of our place in society. Not only do these subconscious beliefs make for a dreadful prospect, but they also make it impossible not to rely on medication to manage the accompanying side-effects.

In Britain, the number of prescriptions issued has risen threefold in just 15 years. It is now quite common for those in their seventies and beyond to be taking half a dozen, and often considerably more, different drugs every day.

---

1 http://www.sciencedaily.com/releases/2013/12/131231094353.htm

WE ARE MORE THAN THE SUM OF OUR PARTS

For most of us health is characterised by the absence of disease and the good functioning of our mind and body. In fact most of us are more familiar with the concept of *ill* health than health. Health is not having to think about it! Yet how can we hope to maintain it if we don't?

THE IMPORTANCE OF INTERACTIONS

There are two fundamental principles on which to build a better understanding of health in order to support it. The first is that, far from a state of being, health is the result of a continuous and dynamic adjustment between our physiology, our environment and our outlook. The second is that it can be defined only in terms of interactions because nothing ever exists in isolation. Our biological systems (circulatory, digestive, nervous, etc) are connected and we are continuously interacting with our environment from the food we eat, the air we breathe, the soap we use, etc to the people we connect with and the information we listen to. To optimise health we have to become more aware of the type of choices we constantly make – and their influence.

It may seem obvious, but life and health are intimately linked and our natural tendency is to thrive. Within every cell are specific preservation mechanisms and within our brain are reward pathways closely associated with pleasure and happiness. The cellular level cannot be dissociated from the whole body and responds directly to the state of mind and attitude of the person, but that doesn't mean that health can be reduced to a state of mind. Our emotional and mental wellbeing is largely dependent on physiological balance and physical comfort; it is very difficult to feel happy when we are hungry, cold or in pain.

No matter how attractive the possibility, health authorities and vast medical bodies cannot take each individual's needs and unique make-up into consideration. When it comes to health, there is no 'one-size fits all'. Because true health can be achieved only at the individual's level, it is our own personal challenge to equip ourselves with properly verified information – even when we have to resort to conventional medical treatment.

Although it is impossible to accurately verify every piece of information, you will find it is health affirming and empowering to become more aware of your dietary and lifestyle choices and some of their possible implications. However, in this age of information technology we are particularly vulnerable to the influence of externally validated truth. It is very easy to accept prescriptive and general recommendations from the medical establishment or the alternative health movement. Typically, each day we hear or read a number of often conflicting 'facts': one source will say 'a healthy diet is the 'Five a day diet', another 'cholesterol is bad' and yet another 'raw vegan food is the only way to achieve vibrant health'. A "System-based" logic is a useful tool to sort through the many contradictory messages that are publicised daily and find a truth that is in harmony with your physiology, your philosophy and your objectives.

THE POWER OF BELIEF

Research in neuroscience and psychology have unequivocally demonstrated the power of belief. So much so, medical trials have to factor placebo in all their 'placebo controlled double-blind studies'. Its effect accounts for up to 30% of results in clinical trials, yet a placebo is not considered a valid medicine. Nonetheless it has to be factored into double blind studies, because simply believing that something is good for us can be enough for lasting reversal of a diseased state. Less obvious, but still influential is the relationship between the health practitioners administering the treatment and their patients. Even more remarkable is the relevance of the belief of the health practitioner about the treatment. This has led researchers to call for triple blind trials in an attempt to keep everybody in the dark. However the sheer impossibility of controlling what a group of people eat, drink, believe, think and act for any length of time while conducting a trial signals the need for thorough systemic referencing within scientific evaluation. The sacrosanct 'double blind study', which falls short of this, makes the pursuit of isolating the effect of a molecule independently from any other relevant factors, essentially flawed. However the placebo is evidence of the power of belief and warns us to be careful with what and whom we choose to believe.

THE EMERGENCE OF SYSTEMIC THINKING

Established medical models such as traditional Chinese medicine, Ayurvedic and naturopathic medicine have a Systemic view of health in common. They were derived over many centuries from observing nature and it is encouraging to see this intuitive understanding finally backed by modern science. For example, research on the function and action of gut bacteria on immunity reveals that certain bacteria will support immunity within specific and variable parameters but only if the equilibrium between organism types is favourable. It is now known and widely accepted that our emotional state influences this equilibrium and this in turn has an impact on our immune system. The variability of the components shows that the outcome lies in the *balance* of the interactions and not in the components themselves. Illness is more likely to be the result of biological retroactive and interactive connections, rather than a direct expression or collection of symptoms with specific causes (such as a disease-causing bacteria, a trauma or a mineral deficiency).

The last 25 years have seen an explosion of research demonstrating the influence of the environment on certain diseases and genetic tendencies. Research in bio-chemistry and nutrition, as well as in microbiology, has shown how the effect of a particular molecule or microbe is never isolated and must be considered in relation to other factors. For example, opposing hormones, such as adrenaline versus nor-adrenaline and insulin versus glucagon, are not the simplistic binary system they were once thought to be. Stress and blood sugar levels are regulated by individual factors and back-up hormones. The specific mode of action and consequences of those hormones are much less predetermined than originally expected. Similarly the highly anticipated human genome research project launched in 1993 has essentially failed to attribute the cause of disease to specific genes and instead revealed that epigenetic (the cofactors arising from non-genetic influences on gene expression) is far more influential in gene expression than the genes themselves.

SEEING THE WOOD AS WELL AS THE TREES: SYSTEMIC ANALYSIS AND THE IMPORTANCE OF INTERACTIONS

Health can be viewed 'systemically' by looking at the overall interactions of its components. This holistic analysis provides a deeper insight into health and the mechanisms which control ageing. It helps create more effective tools to positively rebalance interactions between organs and the nervous and hormonal systems while influencing healthier choices and behaviour.

A systemic analysis of health identifies each element of (human) biology as a defined system. Specific and connected interactions are applicable regardless of the biological system analysed (a cell, an organ, a biological function or a person). They are:

1. Interactions strictly inside the system
2. Interactions strictly outside the system
3. Interactions between the inside and the outside of the system

Those interactions exist whatever the type (simple or complex), the nature (abstract or concrete) or the size (microscopic or macroscopic) of the system

THE 4 BIO-SYSTEMIC LEVELS	APPLIED TO THE INDIVIDUAL	APPLIED TO A CELL
1 Interactions inside the system (state)	Inborn personality (nature)	The entirety of the bio-chemical activities taking place within the cell and which participate in its function
2 Interactions outside the system (environment)	Socio-cultural environment that contextualises the individual (nurture)	The characteristics of the interstitial fluid bathing the cell
3 Interactions at the interface between the inside and the outside of the system (exchange)	Education, social interactions and family dynamics that directly influence individual expression	The activities taking place at the semi-selective cell membrane for the vital exchanges between the cell and its environment
4 The overall consequences (purpose)	The way in which an individual defines his role in society, and the direct consequence of nature, nurture and experience	The specific function of that cell and its genetic expression derived from all the other interactions

and they always have an overall consequence or purpose. Even the interactions that take place outside of the system influence the outcome.

The table (above) shows those three interactive levels and their consequences comparatively applied to the cell and to the individual. This illustrates the patterns and similarities which underline all biological systems and are the foundation of systemic analysis.

This systemic model demonstrate that health is dynamic and the result of constant exchanges and adjustments (interactions) that maintain the equilibrium and purpose of the whole.

BIO-FEEDBACK AND THE RELATIONSHIP BETWEEN FORM AND FUNCTION

Good health is meaningful only if we have a sense of purpose for which we thrive. For an athlete, health is achieving physical goals, for an elderly person being healthy may simply be being pain-free, drug-free and independent. As we age, our objectives and wellbeing goals change. At 30 we want to look good to be attractive to a suitable mate, at 80 we want to live life without a wheelchair. Relationships are just as important but don't carry the same significance. As we age we become more interested in the person we are interacting with than what they look like or their sexual power.

Stem cell technology has developed a process of three-dimensional printing by which each undifferentiated stem-cell is 'informed' of what to build from the shape of a 'printing scaffold'. In so doing, it becomes a specific tissue like a tooth. Similarly if we repeat an action frequently enough our body will adapt to accommodate that action. This could be a positive healthy consequence like stronger bones from weight bearing exercise, or the very opposite such as loss of muscle from anti-gravity as is the case with astronauts or people who are bed-bound.

Mindfulness and the process of becoming aware isn't just a way of managing stress or being more present to our experience, it is also an opportunity to change the outcome. If we are to age well and achieve optimum health we must also commit to making this a reality now.

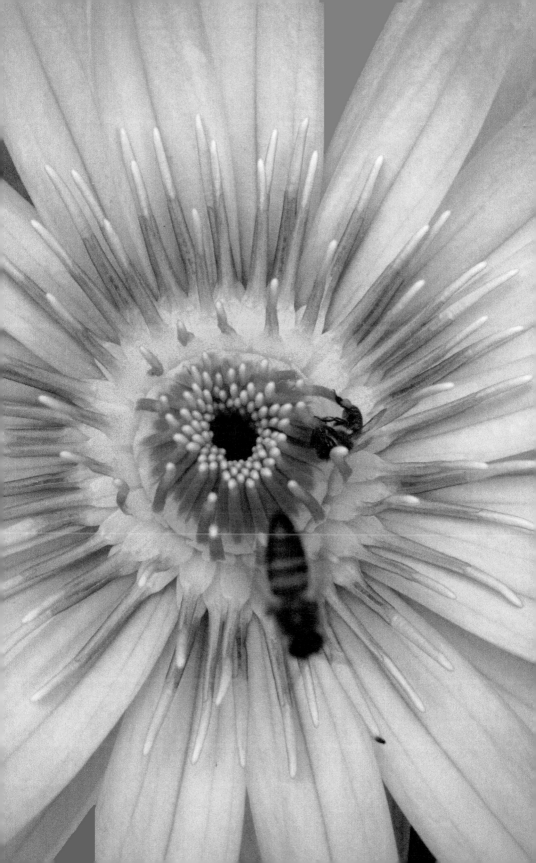

NO MORE 'DIETS'

The *Too Young to Grow Old* programme is made up of simple elements that can be adapted to your own lifestyle. Each element can be managed relative to what is possible even when choices are limited by your work, social or financial situation.

A PROGRAMME THAT CAN EASILY BE ADAPTED TO THE CHALLENGES OF MODERN LIFE

Most of our choices are subconscious; directed by habit, lack of time or misplaced priorities such as preferring fast food over health food. However a large part of our behaviour is also motivated by our physiology. As we change the physiology, the behaviour will change. No matter how small the changes, over time the impact will be cumulative and will feed the desire for more energy, more positive moods, more restful sleep, more confidence, and more stamina. That desire is fed by the glimpses we gather along the way into greater health and wellbeing. Slowly but surely the choices we make evolve and become part of our chosen health path.

FAT IS NOT THE ENEMY

One of the key elements to emerge from recent research on nutrition and obesity is in the significance of the type of fuel that feeds our cells. This can be more, or less efficient, and health promoting, depending if it is fat or sugar. It has long been assumed that glucose is the preferred energy source for our body becasue the brain cannot function without it. This has now been clearly demonstrated not to be the case. The brain can and does function on ketone bodies[1] (an energy source produced from fat) as well as glucose. Ketones are also particularly suited to heart function. In fact the more generally efficient the cells are at fuelling on fat the healthier we become in terms of risk factors for diabetes, heart disease, and many cancers. And of course we become leaner too. There are a number of ways we can improve fat-burning. The more our cells are forced to burn fat the better they become at doing it without the awful feeling associated with blood-sugar dips. Conversely if we never challenge our cells to convert into fat-burning they tend to become inefficient, especially when

---

1 http://www.ncbi.nlm.nih.gov/pubmed/15877199

combined with other factors like genetics. When this happens fat becomes easier to store than to burn. One of the benefits that you will notice from improving your fat-burning ability is how well this makes you feel. Energy levels are more even, thinking clears, cravings become easier to control and emotions less erratic.

THE PLEASURE PRINCIPLE

Awareness of choice is only one side of the coin. If it leads to an obsessional preoccupation with the sensitive nature of our body then we miss a fundamental element of health which is pleasure. Health mustn't be mystified or taken for granted; but understood and enjoyed. Pleasure is essential and helps to balance us mentally.

Our choices and actions may be motivated by ideals, convictions or forces (such as love) but the fact is that human experience requires either pleasure or pain to nudge us into even a small change. While pain is strongly motivating, pleasure is a lot more pleasant and a gentler path, but ultimately both pain and pleasure are intrinsic to our human experience.

Although health is and should be the ultimate pleasure, not all pleasures are healthy. Some behaviours and substances that trigger pleasure have the potential to become addictive. Sugar and alcohol require less effort than exercise to become addictive, but all three hold the same potential.

Addiction develops when the initial pleasure response begins to decrease in intensity and requires ever greater amounts for us to get the same 'high'. Soon after that every other potentially healthy but simple pleasure, such as spending time with friends or appreciating music, becomes bland and unrewarding. However we are much less likely to develop addictions if we fully connect with the pleasure element and consciously choose our pleasures. It's important to be aware that most addictions are a way to escape rather than an uncontrollable need for pleasure.

It is well-known that more than 90% of people fail to keep their New Year resolutions beyond the middle of February because they focus on 'sticking to a programme'. It is a test of willpower which is already in limited supply! Willpower is a very different neurological response to that of pleasure. Pleasure is associated with reward, while willpower is resisting the urge. Have you ever noticed how the mere idea of going on a diet will make you want to binge?

While we are involved with NOT doing something, we are in fact thinking about nothing else so it is a far more effective strategy to think about how we will get rewarded. The anticipation of pleasure and the projection of reward are not just motivating – they are a source of pleasure in themselves.

Pleasure is also a highly therapeutic power, which, if carefully harnessed, makes a huge contribution to our health and wellbeing. Laughter, expressing gratitude, sharing a meal with friends, playing sport, dancing, singing or listening to music, breathing fresh air, cooking and eating fresh and delicious food are pleasures which will enhance our wellbeing and experience of life, as well as enhance immune activity, promote better digestion and reduce stress.

JUNK FOOD IS NEVER A "TREAT": RESISTING MANIPULATION AND THE REWARDS OF SELF-EMPOWERMENT

When I ran a residential training centre, students stayed at my house and were served abundant and delicious vegetable-based dishes. Most of them found the change of diet a challenge and they would fantasise about all the 'treats' they were missing. 'Treats' was a euphemism for chocolate bars, fizzy drinks, wine, hamburgers, French fries and white bread. Of course they knew that these were of no nutritional value and that is precisely why they called them treats! The paradox fascinates me. How can an empty food, commonly referred to as junk, be a treat? I call it an addiction or a poison but not a treat.

To me, this illustrates our vulnerability to manipulation and self-delusion. If advertisements did not so cleverly convince us that junk food is the perfect accompaniment to sex, fun, a successful life and peak fitness we might be less interested. Clearly external influences like advertising have a powerful impact on our behaviour but what of the internal chatter that inhabits our minds?

One of the most significant turning points in my life was when I became aware of the profound influence my 'mind-talk' had on my daily experience and choices. As I realised this I saw how I could influence my choices and behaviour by altering the narrative and turning disempowering internal dialogue into a more supportive conversation. Instead of 'denying' myself 'treats' I thought about the pleasant results of healthy food. In this way junk food was no longer disguised into a treat or pleasure confused with self-destructive bingeing.

Initially this seemed to herald a greater sense of control but I soon realised that freedom and self-empowerment was the reward, not control. Indeed the point of it isn't to replace one (negative) statement with another (positive) one but to gain insight into what actually drives us, so we are less at the mercy of the many limiting messages we receive from advertisers, educators and health professionals, as well as well-meaning family and friends.

To choose freely for ourselves and decide how we want to experience our life requires self-awareness and consciousness of the factors that influence us – even our own minds!

THE FIBRE
FACTOR

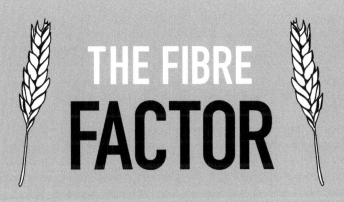

In 60 years the number of overweight people in the UK went from one quarter to one third of the population and is still rising, yet we eat fewer calories, less sugar and less fat than we did in 1950.

Since then, **FIBRE INTAKE PLUMMETED**

from **70g** per day

to barely **20g.**

radically affecting the diversity of our bowel flora.

Could FIBRE be the missing link?

http://www.nutrition.org.uk/attachments/144_Food%20availability%20and%20our%20changing%20diet.pdf

TARGETING METABOLIC STRESSORS AND REVERSING AGEING

The symptoms of ageing are specific to our individual experience, but regardless of personal circumstances we all share the metabolic consequences of stress. In our collective consciousness stress is often limited to an emotional experience such as the loss of a loved one or the fear of looming work targets but there are in fact six types of stress that impact on our physiology in their own way and lead to premature ageing

They are:

- **Mental/emotional stress** which causes nervous exhaustion
- **Nutritional stress** which leads to metabolic dysfunctions and chronic inflammation
- **Toxic stress** which burdens the cells, disrupts hormones and organ function, reduces metabolism and makes us feel confused and sluggish
- **Oxidative stress** which damages DNA and cell integrity and contributes to premature ageing of cells, organs and tissues
- **Lack of movement and interaction with gravity** which impairs neurological and musculoskeletal function
- **Lack of sleep and recovery** which leads to impaired hormonal balance, interference of the appetite hormone, immune disruption and nervous exhaustion

Characteristically 'stress' is needed for us to grow and raise our resistance to it. Popular wisdom has it that "whatever doesn't kill us makes us stronger". Indeed we build muscles by challenging them with the stress of heavy weight and we become better at handling work targets with practice. However a metabolic stressor is not the same as a healthy challenge. Sometimes the difference lies in our attitude and sometimes a healthy challenge becomes a stress because we don't allow sufficient recovery time. Over time metabolic stressors lead to dysfunctions. These will appear before diseases are diagnosed but are not symptom-free. The symptoms are typically associated with (premature) ageing but are in fact the consequence of identified stressors leading to loss of function. They can serve as personal feedback and help assess progress.

The following common symptoms can serve as personal feedback and help assess progress:

- **For mental/emotional stress:** irritability, intolerance, anxiety, lacking in self-confidence, angry, tearful, depressed, 'tired all the time', weight around the middle
- **For malnutrition:** digestive symptoms (pain, bloating, nausea), fatigue, dry skin, dry hair, dull eyes, brittle hair and nails, uneven skin tone, ptosis (lack of

skin tone), acid urine (consistently below Ph6 in the morning and burning)
- **For toxicity:** water retention, difficulty getting up in the morning, fatigue, lack of enthusiasm, allergies, skin rashes, grey looking skin, dark puffy circles under the eyes, dark urine
- **For lack of movement:** low muscle mass, lack of strength, lack of stamina, joint pain, osteoporosis, stiffness, injury, fatigue, weight gain, inflammation, reduced metabolic rate
- **For oxidative stress:** wrinkles, grey complexion, hardening of the arteries, lungs, skin, loss of muscle and tendon elasticity and frequent injuries
- **For poor sleep hygiene:** fatigue, nervousness, depression, appetite dysfunction, cravings, addictions, mental breakdown, sexual dysfunction, reduced immunity and auto-immune disease

If unrectified, metabolic dysfunctions will slowly lead to the cellular breakdown that underlies premature ageing and eventually disease. In the majority of cases this will be a slow and gradual process of repetitive and cumulative stresses. For instance, it is hypothesised that it takes seven to eight years for cancer cells to form a tumour. This gradual loss of cell coherence is sensitive and can be more easily reversed earlier in the process. Once disease has set in, medication becomes more critical to avoid irreversible damage but its effect can add to the metabolic burden that contributed to the disease. The fact that cancer treatments are in themselves carcinogenic and anti-depressants can cause depression[2] illustrates this paradox and makes supporting your health a priority. Conventional medicine doesn't know how to care for health, it only ever controls the symptoms of disease.

Occasionally a functional imbalance can appear suddenly, perhaps after a shock (loss of a loved one, or divorce), an accident (car crash or a fall), surgery, a serious infection (viral, bacterial, and parasitic) or exposure to high levels of toxins (chemotherapy, anaesthetic, antibiotics, carbon monoxide, chemical fumes, and pesticides from field-spray). In this case damage may be more profound and symptoms more severe. Recovery may take longer but will still benefit from a holistic approach because the way in which someone expresses the effect of that trauma is unique to them and the product of all the complex relationships that exist between their constitution and circumstances.

HEALTH IS MORE THAN SKIN DEEP

A revealing study[3] conducted in 2007 on 4025 American women aged between 40 and 74 concluded that diet is more effective than cosmetic surgery to improve skin appearance. On average, the women who consumed a diet rich

2 http://www.psychologytoday.com/blog/mad-in-america/201106/now-antidepressant-induced-chronic-depression-has-name-tardive-dysphoria]
3 http://www.ncbi.nlm.nih.gov/pubmed/17921406

in antioxidants and low in anti-nutrients (sugar, fried foods etc) looked 10.4 years younger than their biological age. Cosmetic surgery could acheive only an 8.9 years average reduction. The study reached those conclusions by measuring the depth and number of wrinkles, by assessing the dryness of the skin and by comparing atrophy of the subcutaneous tissue.

My approach to health and rejuvenation is aimed at reducing cellular ageing through dietary and lifestyle strategies specifically designed to control oxidative stress, toxicity and chronic inflammation. Cell damage can be limited, and sometimes even reversed. Simple lifestyle and dietary measures will benefit your general health but target the skin[4] and general appearance in particular in the following ways:

- Optimum amounts of quality micro-nutrients (antioxidants, vitamins, trace elements, essential fatty acids and amino acids) nourish the skin and tissues.
- A diet rich in antioxidants and trace nutrients contributes to a clear complexion, preserves skin integrity, protects against sun radiation and oxidative damage from pollution.
- Better elimination targeting the liver, bowel, kidneys, lungs and skin reduces metabolic poisons linked to DNA damage and cellular ageing. An accumulation of toxins leads to swelling, puffiness, low metabolism, hormonal disruption and cellulite.
- Improved digestive health, gut lining function and intestinal ecology reduce chronic inflammation. Studies have shown reduced skin hyper-sensitivity (irritation, redness and acute reaction to cold or dry atmospheres) from improved bowel ecology and supplementation with specific probiotics.
- Intermittent fasting stimulates overall detoxification and elimination of damaged cells. It has been shown to positively reduce acne, psoriasis and skin inflammation.
- A diet low in sugar controls low grade inflammation and improves immunity; a low sugar diet has been shown[5] to reduce the number of acne lesions.
- Better strategies to manage emotional stress. Stress shuts down peripheral circulation and disrupts hormonal balance, leading to accelerated ageing.
- Improved human growth hormone status through exercise improves skin tone and elasticity and fat-to-muscle ratio. Exercise improves skin appearance, counteracts stress hormones and stimulates peripheral circulation.
- Selected skin care products protect the skin and limit exposure to potentially toxic ingredients. The skin has been shown to absorb large molecules such as the preservative paraben, extensively used in skincare products and known to be a carcinogen[6].

4 http://www.ncbi.nlm.nih.gov/pmc/articles/PMC2836433
5 http://www.ncbi.nlm.nih.gov/pmc/articles/PMC2836431
6 http://www.ncbi.nlm.nih.gov/pubmed/25128701

MY AGE-DEFYING HEALTH PROGRAMME

Based on six complementary aspects of health, my age defying programme combines the following life-enhancing elements:

Raised mental awareness to deal effectively with mental and emotional stress. This is discussed in Part 2.

Re-enforced health/pleasure mental connections to encourage healthier choices and behaviour. In Part 2 you will find a further explanation as to why pleasure is linked to self-empowerment and is impossible to achieve without (self)awareness/mindfulness.

Specific detoxification protocols to activate the mechanisms of cellular preservation. We are more than ever exposed to toxic chemicals and poisons. In Part 3 you will find tried and tested ways to effectively counteract this increasing burden.

Optimised bowel flora to help support the delicate entente cordiale that exists between our trillions of gut bacteria and our immune, neurological and digestive health. In Part 3 you will also find ways to improve and capitalise on the precious "friendly bacteria" that inhabit the bowel.

Increased fat-burning to reduce chronic inflammation and slow tissue ageing. Discover in Part 3 simple ways to train your body to burn fat instead of sugar.

Targeted nutrition to create lasting health. In Part 4 you will find 'The 10 Principles of Choice' – my general dietary recommendations for lasting health and age reversal.

Practical ways of putting the above into practice are covered in Part 5 (menu planners) and Part 6 (recipes).

MEASURING UP

The explosion across the world of the chronic diseases which tend to affect people as they get older, such as diabetes, Alzheimer's disease, atherosclerosis, arthritis, obesity and cancer, has meant that they have been the object of extensive scientific studies connecting premature ageing with chronic inflammation. Current thinking is definitely evolving towards a more global understanding of the factors involved in chronic inflammation. These are targeted by my programme and are:

- Malnutrition, deficiencies of essential nutrients and imbalance between the major essential fatty acids
- Toxicity and poor elimination
- Metabolic dysfunction and insulin resistance
- Sedentary lifestyle and adrenal stress
- Oxidative stress from free radicals
- Gut dysbiosis - an imbalance of microbia in the digestive tract

Research has demonstrated relationships between gut inflammation and mental health (not just neurotransmitter deficiency), and between insulin resistance and lack of exercise (not just genetic or caused by diet as previously thought). It is rapidly becoming clear that even apparently remote connections exist. Therefore to restore better health and reverse chronic disease we must apply a coherent and integrated approach.

It is also becoming apparent that chronic diseases are starting earlier in life with an increasing number of young adults suffering from diabetes, and early onset Alzheimer's or dementia. The latter has now overtaken cancer in a recent survey of most feared diseases[7]. Although we live a lot longer than our ancestors, the degenerative process of ageing is starting younger and leading to an increasing number of years on medication and in poor health.

By definition a chronic disease is managed with medication but not cured, and will tend to have a very slow but fairly predictable prognosis despite prescribed treatment and drugs.

---

7 https://www.metlife.com/assets/cao/contributions/foundation/alzheimers-2011.pdf

Chronic diseases are characterised by the following symptoms:

- Obesity
- Depression
- Digestive problems (IBS, acid reflux, ulcers, constipation etc)
- Hormonal imbalance and menopausal symptoms
- Stress, anxiety and depression
- Auto-immune disease (Hashimoto, MS, Crohn's, Parkinson's disease etc)
- Chronic pain, restricted movement, stiffness and arthritis
- Alzheimer's disease
- Cardiovascular diseases
- Insulin resistance (syndrome X) and diabetes.
  Syndrome X is medically characterised by two or more of the following symptoms:
  - ✓ Waist circumference greater than 40 inches (for men) and 36 inches (for women)
  - ✓ Triglyceride levels greater than 150 mg/dL (1.69mmol/L)
  - ✓ Fasting glucose greater than 100 mg/dL (5.6 mmol/L)
  - ✓ A fasting serum insulin level greater than 25 ml U/L (174 pmol/L)
  - ✓ Blood pressure greater than 130/85
  - ✓ HDL lower than 40, and LDL greater than 100

These syndromes and types of symptoms are also a measurement of health and a marker of our physiological age. They serve as a way to evaluate progress and their severity should alert us to the urgency to modify our diet, lifestyle and mental state in order to avoid the predictable degradation that comes from chronic disease.

Frequently my chronic disease patients will report asking their consultant or GP about the benefits of altering their diet. Depending on their particular condition the answers range from: "it will make no difference", to outdated and standard dietary restrictions such as avoiding so called cholesterol-raising foods, or eating a diet of processed foods devoid of fibre – in the case of severe diarrhoea

Although there has been plenty of research on the implication of diet on various disease states, hardly any of the more recent findings have trickled down to actual recommended medical guidelines. The research protocols themselves can reduce and limit scientific studies to isolated elements, making it difficult to translate them into a coherent diet that is applicable to real people. As a result dietary factors are still regarded as irrelevant to disease by the majority of Western medical practitioners.

BLOOD TESTS AND MEASURING PROGRESS

Setting up targets and measuring progress is essential when undergoing any change, otherwise why would you want to keep the changes? And how would you know that something positive is happening?

Although the symptoms mentioned above are accurate measurements they can also be correlated with some basic blood tests. To have blood tests done regularly is useful because they can reveal metabolic changes regardless of symptoms. They help set up targets and the results can prove more immediate and motivating than a set of scales or a measuring tape. I recommend that you speak to your general practitioner to establish the levels of the following health markers: fasting blood glucose, triglycerides, uric acid and C reactive protein (CRP).

The levels considered acceptable by your GP are likely to be different from those I will give you. This is because the references used for the medical range are based on an average among the general population which may be disease-free but not always healthy.

Rather than reassure us that we are 'normal' (meaning average) the blood tests should help us establish a metabolic trend and indicate how successful we are with the programme and principles outlined in this book. **You need to start measuring and comparing your own personal levels.**

Fasting Blood Sugar

According to **medical standards,** normal fasting blood glucose is below 100 mg/dL (5.6 mmol/L). A person with a fasting blood glucose level between 110 mg/dL (6.1 mmol/L) and 125 mg/dL (6.9 mmol/L) is considered pre-diabetic and if the level rises to 126 mg/dL (7.00 mmol/L) or above, they are diagnosed with full-blown diabetes.

However when testing fasting blood sugar on people who are healthy and paying attention to their diet the number drops to 85/87 mg/dL (4.7/4.8 mmol/L) and even reaches 80 mg/dL (4.4 mmol/L) for those who follow more strictly the recommendations for a fat-burning metabolism I discuss in Part 3.

If your fasting blood sugar is between 90 mg/dL (5.00 mmol/L) and 110 mg/dL (6.1mmol/L) you should consider this to be an indication that your metabolism is not efficient at burning fat and is overly dependent on sugar. Your target is to take it slightly below 90 mg/dL (5.00 mmol/L).

Triglycerides

This test is typically done when your cholesterol level is taken. It is important that this test is done after a ten hour fast. One can drink water but no food

should be consumed. The American Heart Association defines the following:
- Normal triglycerides = less than 150 mg/dL (1.69 mmol/L)
- Borderline high triglycerides = 155-320 mg/dL (1.7-2.25 mmol/L)
- High triglycerides = 320-480mg/dL (2.26-5.42 mmol/L)
- Very high triglycerides = higher than 480 mg/dL (5.42 mmol/L)

However a far better triglyceride reading would be below 105 mg/dL (1.20 mmol/L) as evidence of cardiovascular damage is visible even with numbers below 151 mg/dL (1.70 mmol/L). This was corroborated by a recently published study[8] spanning over 30 years which showed that childhood triglyceride levels above 135 mg/dL (1.50 mmol/L) could predict cardiovascular risks in later life.

Uric Acid

Dr Richard Johnson, chief of the division of kidney disease and hypertension at the University of Colorado, has conducted research indicating that there is a proportional connection between uric acid and the body's signalling to store fat. He postulates that the pre-diabetic state is only a natural response to the high sugar/high fructose diet which our ancestors would have had in the autumn before the food restrictions of winter. Nowadays abundance in sugar is never followed by caloric restriction so the body never has a chance to normalise and instead disease ensues.

With this in mind uric acid levels are not just indicative of a predisposition to the pain of gout but an alarm bell for disrupted metabolism and excessive sugar consumption. What is regarded as normal reading varies from lab to lab. This alone is rather suspicious but generally it will vary along these lines:

Male mg/dL	Female mg/dL
2.10 to 8.50	2.00 to 7.00

In accordance with Dr Johnson's views I would suggest that the ideal uric acid levels are:

Male mg/dL	Female mg/dL
2.10 to 4.00	2.00 to 3.50

8 http://www.ncbi.nlm.nih.gov/pubmed/19501856

C-Reactive Protein (C-RP)

Baseline levels of C-reactive protein appear to predict future risk of symptomatic peripheral vascular disease, atherosclerosis and secondary clots.

C-reactive protein is also known to be a marker for systemic inflammation. This is very significant because chronic inflammation is now well documented as being the slow burning fire associated with tissue damage and chronic diseases from Alzheimer's, diabetes, cardiovascular risk, depression, auto-immune diseases and arthritis. C-RP levels that are associated with low cardiovascular risk and reflect positively on chronic inflammation are less than 1.0 mg/L. levels must be tested when there are no current known causes of inflammation such as an injury or an infection. **An acceptable range is 1.0 to 3.0 mg/L.** Levels above that should alert you to a state of underlying chronic inflammation and the need to follow the stricter guidelines in Part Three for reducing chronic inflammation.

Gamma Glutamyl Transpeptidase (gamma-G-T)

A liver enzyme involved in detoxification and a good liver function marker. The lower the better but **should be less than 40 IU/L.**

Alanine Aminotransferase (ALT)

Another liver enzyme also involved in detoxification.

The normal range is less than 40 U/L but according to Dr Robert Lustig (an American paediatric endocrinologist and author of *Fat Chance: The Hidden Truth about Sugar, Obesity and Disease*) 25 can already predict a fatty liver.

Fatty liver is associated with metabolic dysfunction. It used to be found mostly among alcoholics but with the increase in the incidence of metabolic dysfunction and diabetes, it is now common in young people who rarely drink alcohol.

OTHER USEFUL MEASUREMENTS

Waist Circumference

As a generally agreed guideline, your waist measurement should be less than than your hip measurement and less than 101cm (40 inches) for men and 91cm (36 inches) for women.

Waist circumference is a good indication of intra-abdominal fat and can safely be a couple of inches below those measurements. Waist circumference is a better way to keep an eye on your "weight" than your actual weight because muscles weigh considerably more than fat.

Body Fat Percentage

Unlike Body Mass Index (BMI), measuring your waist size and your body fat percentage are far more accurate methods to determine whether you are at risk of weight-related health problems like heart disease and diabetes. Fat percentage can be measured with a specialised electronic scale.

It is perfectly possible to have a low to normal body weight but a high fat-to-muscle ratio, and conversely to have an elevated BMI and a low body fat percentage.

	Women (% fat)	Men (%fat)
Essential Fat	10-13%	2-5%
Athletes	14-20%	6-13%
Fitness	21-24%	14-17%
Acceptable	25-31%	18-24%
Obese	32% and higher	25% and higher

Blood Pressure

There is perhaps too much emphasis placed on blood pressure because it varies significantly depending on situation, time of day and equipment used to measure. However a consistently **elevated blood pressure (above 150/90)** when correlated with the above measurements is undoubtedly a cardio vascular risk factor. Lowering the BP without addressing the causes is only partially successful at preventing cardiovascular risks.

In my experience, blood pressure will almost always normalise when addressing the diet and lifestyle elements underlying the condition. Following my recommendations about mental wellbeing, exercise and diet will support a healthy blood pressure and minimise the need for medication.

Celebrating Progress

As the above measurements improve you'll notice a reduction in your symptoms. What tends to happen is that we forget pain as it becomes no longer relevant and remember only the symptoms that are still current. After a couple of weeks of training at the gym you may be sleeping better, feeling less anxious and emptying your bowel every morning **BUT** the weight hasn't shifted yet…this doesn't mean that the ideas behind the programme don't work, it simply means that there is more of it to build into your life.

What makes my approach different from others, is that it is more about a health style than lifestyle and more of a philosophy than a specific anti-ageing programme.

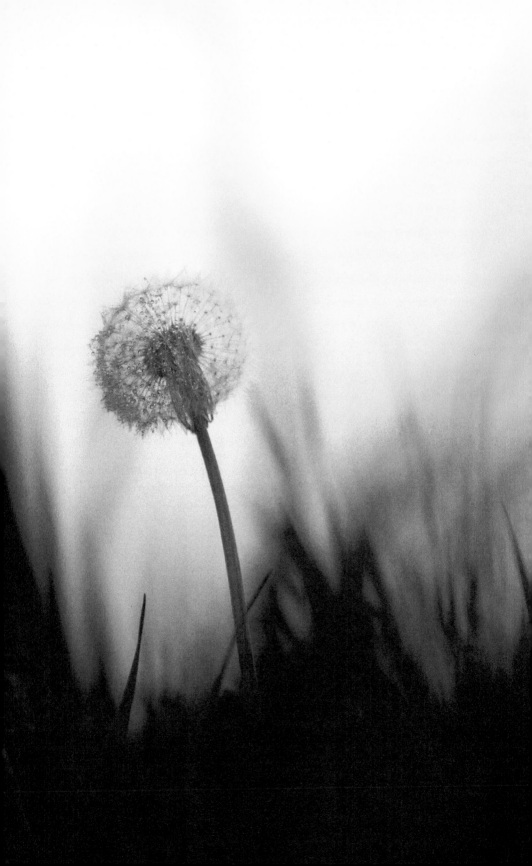

PART TWO:
CHECK INTO THE
STRESS CLINIC

"A thought which does not result in an action is nothing much, and an action which does not proceed from a thought is nothing at all."

GEORGE BERNANOS

BREAKING FREE WITH MINDFULNESS

Stress is perhaps the greatest contributor to ageing. It increases cortisol levels, which are directly implicated in belly fat; it disrupts metabolism, causes anxiety, contributes to chronic inflammation and generally speeds up cellular ageing. Everyone knows that stress is very damaging to health and entire books are devoted to the subject of stress management.

Yet the very notion that stress can be managed, treated or even cured reduces it to a symptom for which there must be a remedy – such as deep breathing or meditation. Relaxation techniques are beneficial for the symptoms, but we need to look at the causes.

A different way to look at it would be to say that stress is the consequence of several mental and physiological factors, all of which are inter-connected but no single item is the actual cause. Stepping back and viewing ourselves systemically opens up positive ways to influence our stress response. Instead of making us sick and old we can use stress positively. In this chapter we will look at how to turn it around to keep us healthy and young.

THE CONSEQUENCE OF PHYSIOLOGY

Our physiology is not independent from our stress response; it is obviously affected by stress but it also drives it. We all have experienced a dry mouth or faster heartbeat when faced with a stressful situation. This is the natural response to perceived or real danger and primes us to fight or flee. If we are already in a state of chronic low-grade stress we will be even more sensitive and rapidly cumulate the effects into a 'chronic stress physiology'. Significant stressors that contribute to this state include lack of sleep, smoking, sugar and intake of stimulants. Even allergies and food sensitivities can drive an immune modulated stress response. The healthier we are the more resistant we can be to the cumulative effects of stress. However our personality also plays a major part in how we deal with stressful situations and understanding our personality requirements alongside simple diet and lifestyle adjustments can bring lasting and significant results.

THE INFLUENCE OF PERSONALITY

The work of Professor Robert Sapolsky, a neuro-endocrinologist, professor of neuroscience and neurosurgery at Stanford University, on stress and attitude is most inspiring. In particular he tells the story of a tribe of baboons[1] in Kenya that he studied extensively over a couple of decades. When he began observing them, the social order of the tribe was a classic hierarchal structure based around the dominant males maintaining their status by regularly chastising females, and bullying lesser males who in turn, bullied still lesser males.

This went on for years until the tribe was decimated by tuberculosis. The baboons which survived the epidemic were at the bottom of the social ladder, and not involved in bullying nor concerned about maintaining their place in the social hierarchy. Their immune resistance was attributed to lower levels of stress and stress hormones, but what is even more interesting is that they went on to breed a completely different tribe with no dominating individuals bullying their way to the top. Instead they were all involved with supporting each other, demonstrating this by grooming, sharing and generally being kind to one another. This is an unusual social order for a baboon community and it illustrates the interconnection between nurture and nature. If applied to the human experience it demonstrates that a naturally less aggressive nature nurtured to be gentle will continue to breed that characteristic. A state of constant alertness will breed stress induced and aggressive behaviour that will perpetuate stress for ourselves and those around us.

Clearly our personality plays a major role in the frustration, anxiety and restlessness usually associated with stress. If personality hinders our ability to choose, then a systemic look at personality and the interactions between each of the building blocks that make up our emotional stability and self-esteem will bring greater freedom to choose.

When we are connected with our power to make choices instead of feeling out of control and permanently threatened and influenced by the physiological consequences, we feel calmer – even if faced with a difficult situation.

Unless there is real danger, an unpleasant encounter is never life-threatening, but can be damaging to our ego. Understanding how our personality functions and the triggers that threaten our self-esteem is an empowering way to control stress, because it recognises that it is within our power to change our response.

Using the **4 interactive levels analysis**, a systemic view of the building blocks of our personality may look like this:

---

[1] A Primate's Memoir: A Neuroscientist's Unconventional Life Among the Baboons by Robert M. Sapolsky

THE 4 INTERACTIVE LEVELS	APPLIED TO PERSONALITY
1 Interactions inside the system (state)	• Personality driven needs for: significance, variety, certainty and connection with others • Multiple innate factors that shape our personality (including innate personality factors and genetic influences)
2 Interactions outside the system (environment)	• Education, parental influence and significant other's influence • Cultural, religious and media influence • Acquired factors that shape our personality (including commensal gut microbe, childhood vaccinations, diet, lifestyle, diseases, pollutants etc)
3 At the interface between the two	• The interpretation of the experiences that form our personality and are the product of our innate tendencies and acquired imprinting
4 The overall purpose	• Awareness • Growth, self-knowledge and learning • Choice • Freedom from personality demands

This table highlights the considerable variety of factors that shape our personality. It also shows the necessity to keep in mind the overall purpose for greater freedom from the tyranny of our ego, so that we can apply choice and grow as healthy individuals. It is said that our greatest gift, and what distinguishes us from animals, is **choice**, a direct consequence of consciousness.

The next section seeks to give an empowering perspective on the mental patterns and personality needs that influence our responses from **stress-able** to **response-able.** It gives various tools that are designed to increase self-awareness. They are founded in the assertion that harmony between choices, core values, behaviour and self beliefs support health and happiness. Conversely, the discomfort and malaise associated with stress, anxiety and depression are simply there to alert us to the discord between those elements.

MICROBES GET

STRESSED TOO

···

PSYCHOLOGICAL STRESS

SUPPRESSES

BENEFICIAL BACTERIA

IN THE GUT.

The stools of university students have been shown to contain fewer beneficial lactobacillus at exam time than at the relatively trouble-free beginning of term.

http://www.apa.org/monitor/2012/09/gut-feeling.aspx

CHOICE IS OUR MOST POWERFUL ASSET

Every day, several times a day, we are making choices that are liable to impact on how we feel, yet only occasionally do we consider the consequences. In fact we are rarely conscious that we are *choosing* anything much at all. We follow mental patterns and habits that are the results of repetition.

We are constantly confronted by situations that require making choices, but we rarely know what exactly makes us choose an item on a menu or adopt a particular interpretation of what someone says. To improve health we must become conscious of the fact that we are making choices and then develop awareness of the physical and mental effects of those choices.
Only in this way can we:
- **Develop** experience and knowledge about the mechanisms that motivate our choices
- **Change** an acquired habitual (stress) response into a healthy mindful choice
- **Become** wiser about the true impact an individual choice has on the way we feel
- **Make** lasting meaningful changes that contribute to our health. Each of us is the product of a society, a culture, a family, an education – and a personality. We have beliefs and values that are passed down to us in the same way as we inherit our DNA. As social primates, our innate tendency is to submit to the influence of authority such as government, teachers and the media, and our natural inclination is to follow the herd. Awareness of *how* we select a lifestyle choice or a core value frees us from habitually repeating an acquired behaviour or following 'common sense' (sometimes 'individual sense' might be a better choice!). Awareness brings individuality to the fore and connects us with our own needs.

The two diagrams on the following pages show how we lean towards a reactive behavioural pattern or informed choice and self-empowerment.
In the first illustration we see confusion arises when we are restricted by a combination of useless or contradictory information, an overly critical mind and poorly defined aims. In the second illustration we see that change is conditional upon self-responsibility, a fruitful aim and useful information.

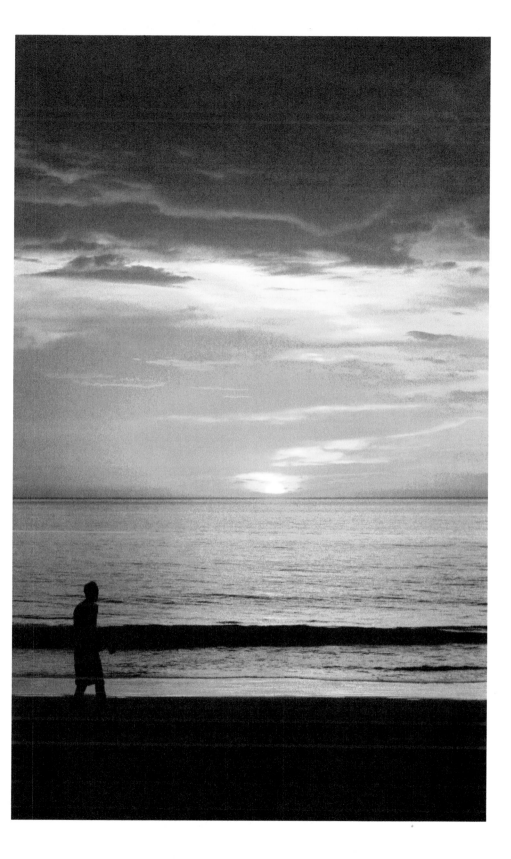

UNABLE TO CHANGE AND LEARN

When we are in 'stress' mode we react without awareness and we are unable to change and to learn.

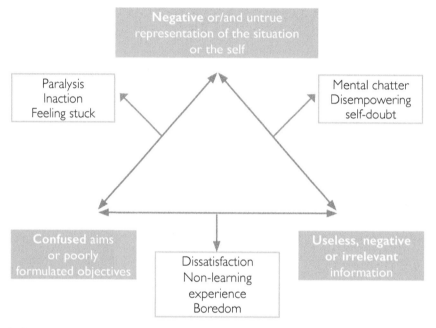

When we have a desire to create change, or when we want to be clearer about our objectives, but are feeling unable to put our desire for change into action the following questions can help identify how we have become stuck or can simply give us direction:

- What are my goals and are they defined in a positive way? eg. What I *aim* to achieve, rather than what I don't want to do?
- What specific information will help me achieve my goals and how am I going to obtain that information?
- Is my assessment of the current situation based on an objective evaluation, or repeating habitual patterns and following negative beliefs about myself?
- Is my current behaviour in accordance with my goal, or am I sabotaging my intent and efforts?

SELF-EMPOWERMENT

When we are mindful we are conscious of our choices and able to create positive actions towards change. This will result in self-empowerment from the following interactions:

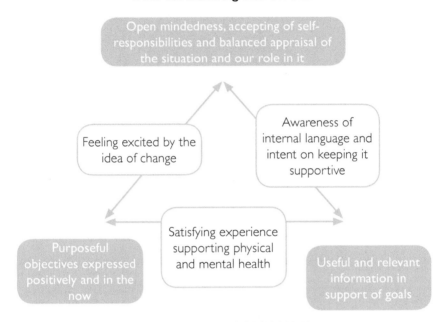

Open mindedness, accepting of self-responsibilities and balanced appraisal of the situation and our role in it

Feeling excited by the idea of change

Awareness of internal language and intent on keeping it supportive

Purposeful objectives expressed positively and in the now

Satisfying experience supporting physical and mental health

Useful and relevant information in support of goals

INCREASE YOUR CAPACITY TO ADAPT AND RESIST STRESS BY:

- **Regularly challenging your habits:** walk a different way to the shop, sit in a different chair, move furniture around, experiment with foods. Ensure that you are comfortable with the idea of minor and frequent change.
- **Practising mindfulness and self-awareness (however uninteresting the task):** learn to be aware in a situation of your bodily sensations, your surroundings and the people around you. Be mindful when you walk or exercise and also when you eat, listen to a friend tell her story, or wait for the bus. These daily opportunities connect with your life's experience instead of seeking distraction from it. Smart phones are the distraction of choice these days and the enemy of mindfulness!
- Be selective and conscious about the information you choose to listen to: eg: the newspaper you read or don't read, the television you watch or don't watch, the friends you hang out with or the subjects you are studying

BEWARE OF EXPECTATIONS

Frequently our awareness stops with an uncomfortable feeling such as anger, frustration, sadness or anxiety, or an incoherent behaviour such as being late, forgetful or lazy. Our natural inclination is to find a way to modify the discomfort rather than sit with it for long enough to understand the deeper causes. For some the answer can be comfort eating, drinking, smoking, or taking drugs; for others it will be a violent expression of anger, or it might be a quiet and repetitive expression of regrets. In reality the discomfort, behaviour and associated emotions all alert us that we are in "stress" mode but they also point out to the need to review our underlying expectations. If we didn't expect others to behave in a certain way we wouldn't get angry when they don't, and if we didn't assume responsibility for what cannot be changed, we wouldn't feel regretful. How we evaluate and assess a situation can either empower us, or on the contrary, externalise the causes of our discomfort to such an extreme that it leaves us with no option for action or change. If we didn't assume responsibility for what cannot be changed, we wouldn't feel regretful. Expectations can only reinforce a sense of failure and are not to be confused with actual goals or objectives.

NEGATIVE AND DISEMPOWERING FEELINGS EXPRESS THEMSELVES:

♦ **At work and in relation to social status:**
  - I have missed my career opportunities
  - It is too late, I am too old now, I will never get out of this situation
  - I am not achieving enough for my career advancement, I am stuck
  - Compared to my colleagues I am not good enough, intelligent enough
  - Everything will be better on holiday
  - I will be more secure once I have achieved X Y Z
  - I am exploited and far too good for this job
  - What's the point?

♦ **In our social interactions:**
  - I am misunderstood
  - Nobody appreciates me, nobody loves me
  - I am the one that always sacrifices everything
  - I am not good enough
  - I am too impatient with my children/partner
  - My children are not achieving enough
  - I deserve a better partner, kinder, sexier…

♦ **In our self-expression and creativity:**
- I am too old or too lacking in talent to take on a creative pursuit such as art, singing or writing
- I have no time for a hobby, exercise or meditation
- Only selfish people take on hobbies, it's more important to be with your family
- My family needs me too much, I can't take time away from them

In our health and lifestyle management:
- I don't have time to eat well, go to the gym, shop for fresh food
- To watch TV while eating a take-away is my favourite treat
- Sugar makes me feel happy and healthy food is boring
- Wine at night helps me sleep
- Smoking helps me think and relax
- Those who look after their bodies are narcissistic
- Exercise is tiring – and dangerous if you are not used to it
- It is too late now to become healthier
- Sleep is less important than computer games or finishing that report
- To lose weight you have to deprive yourself and be prepared for a lot of cravings and hunger pangs

OBJECTIVES CAN BE CONFUSING BECAUSE:

They are expressed in a contradictory fashion (e.g. I want to lose weight but I don't want to change my diet)

Often we like the idea of change but our motivation isn't that strong. Our natural tendency is to resist change; but change comes about when we are motivated by pain, fear or desire. If we don't feel any one of those deeply enough to make significant changes, it is probably not a goal but an expectation from others (or our internal chattering judge) that we should change.

They are unachievable

It may seem obvious that aiming for an unachievable goal is setting ourselves up for failure, but it is what we do when we expect too much of ourselves. Instead of feeling encouraged by our achievements we are constantly measuring and reinforcing failure. In theory the goal might be achievable but in reality it requires so much willpower that we just can't sustain the effort and simply fail.

They are expressed negatively

Even if our goal is positive, the way we express it is important. For instance we may choose to exercise regularly in order to avoid the use of a Zimmer frame in old age. This is motivating healthy behaviour but it is also reinforcing fear every time we go to the gym – instead of creating a positive healthy and fully mobile image of ourselves now and in our old age.

They are based on the assumption that we have unlimited time
Procrastination has all the elements of achievement; it feels and tastes like success, but it hasn't started yet. Whatever goal we set ourselves it is important to understand that it starts here and now…not tomorrow morning, not after the weekend and not when we have achieved some other goal!

INFORMATION CAN BE CONTRADICTORY OR USELESS TO OUR OVERALL PURPOSE

It is impossible to question every bit of information that comes our way, but researching significant decisions will ensure that we are committed and the result will be positively influenced by that commitment. In my experience, coherence of belief is more significant to our health and wellbeing than truth, and a lot easier to establish. There is a difference however between filtering information that supports only a particular belief or prejudice, and keeping an open mind about changing it!

The internet is an awesome tool to spread and enhance human knowledge but it's also a source of unverified and poorly substantiated ideas that requires rigorous analysis. Television is a powerful medium for sending out publicity and ideas, but can those messages be trusted when they are so obviously at the service of governments, multinationals – and of a public that is seeking entertainment? Information is everywhere but is it serving us well? Or does it simply keep us distracted?

Cholesterol is a typical example of how mass media messages are rarely at the service of our health or our intelligence. Cholesterol, which is found in bile, is a vital substance and an important precursor molecule for vitamin D and all steroid hormones (including the adrenal gland hormones). Yet common media-driven knowledge is that cholesterol is generally bad, to the extent that doctors tell their patients to fear it in natural foods like eggs and oysters. Pharmaceutical companies are keen for governments to support their cholesterol-busting drugs (Statins) and will go to great lengths to seduce GPs and medical advisers to prescribe them *en masse*.

Meanwhile the makers of cholesterol-lowering yoghurts will take advantage of the general confusion and market their products by reinforcing the idea that processed dairy products are "healthy" because they can lower cholesterol. The public-health damaging consequence of this coordinated (but warped) information campaign is that most people are convinced that cholesterol (and fat) must be tracked down and eradicated from their diet; eggs become highly suspicious and low fat "probiotic yoghurts" extremely attractive despite their sugar content.

Ultimately, mindfulness and personal responsibility about our choices give us freedom to respond to a situation creatively. In this way "I am misunderstood and suffering from stress" can become "I am dissatisfied with my current situation but I have the possibility to modify my behaviour and my responses. I can address my specific personality needs and look for information that will support me. My satisfaction is my responsibility; my health is my priority." Although the latter will require effort it carries hope and self-empowerment.

BEWARE COMMON TRAPS

Whatever the situation, our objectives and our personality, there are certain patterns and triggers that lure us away from achieving our goals or, at the very least, make the journey more difficult and slow us down.

Moving away from something is not a goal. To move away from our usual habits and patterns without deciding what to put in their place will not sustain us for very long. "I will not shout at my children in this way ever again" is not a goal. "Next time they ignore my request to stop fighting, I will separate them and talk to each one individually" is a goal.

Reiterating our need for change is not the same as changing. Wishing for change is not a commitment and doesn't achieve goals. It only reinforces the distance between where we are now and where we want to go. To make a goal motivating we have to make it a reality by writing it down and specifically talking about it. A lot of people confuse the desire for change with an actual goal. In this way they waste a lot of energy by not changing. They might swing from one extreme lifestyle to another, hopping on and off the latest diet but never managing to keep the weight off or simply be happy with the size they are. Conversely, few people have precise goals and objectives in their lives and fewer still write them down. Dare to be different!

Not all of us are motivated by the same things and in the same way but there are common techniques that help us succeed.

THE FOLLOWING ARE POINTS TO BEAR IN MIND WHEN SETTING OUT GOALS:

• **Goals must be compatible with our values:** "I will work hard and earn enough money to buy a sports car" is not motivating if you care about pollution.
• **Desire, pleasure and passion are more motivating than fear:** Even if what we try to achieve is an effort, the accomplishment is a pleasure. The more we connect with that pleasure the less the effort of the journey will hold us

back. By getting in touch with the physical sensation and emotional satisfaction we associate with achieving our goals we already make it a reality. To visualise our goal of feeling healthy, full of energy and pain-free starts the physical process of our recovery; unlike the fear of losing our battle against an illness (which only goes to make us more aware of it). It is well-documented that our physiology literally changes depending on our attitude and state of mind in relation to hope versus fear.

• **Goals must be broken down into manageable steps to be achievable:** This is perhaps obvious but something that we forget to do when setting a particular target. It's easy to get carried away and focus on what we want to achieve to the detriment of the smaller, and perhaps less exciting, steps in between. Think of running a marathon: only when we train regularly, set objectives of smaller distances and allow time to build up stamina can we ever hope to achieve it.

- **Discipline is the foundation of any goal: In the words of Zig Ziglar**[2] "It was character that got us out of bed, commitment that moved us into action and discipline that enabled us to follow through."

- **Reward makes discipline motivating (and acceptable):** Planning and building in rewards are also useful ways to acknowledge achievements.

- **Success breeds success:** minimising set-backs and reinforcing the benefits we are already enjoying from being on the road to achieving our objectives keeps us heading in that direction. Ultimately there is no other goal.

REVERTING TO TYPE UNDER STRESS AND THE STRESS-TRIGGERS BEST AVOIDED

Aside from life events that we can neither predict nor control, and the emotional triggers that alert us of our reactive (stress-induced) mental state, there are specific physical triggers which also drive our behaviour in unhealthy and disempowering ways. Their predictable (physiological) effects will stimulate cravings and addictive tendencies so avoid these as much as possible:

✓ **Lack of sleep** decreases levels of the satiety hormone (leptin) and increases those of the appetite stimulating hormone (ghrelin). A study[3] estimated that young subjects who had slept less than five hours for two nights running had 18% less leptin and 28% more ghrelin than when they slept for at least six hours. Another study[4] confirmed that subjects who follow a low-calorie diet but regularly sleep less than five and a half hours a night, lose up to 55% less abdominal fat than those who follow a similar eating regime but sleep more than five and a half hours a night.

✓ **Lack of day light exposure** impairs the pineal gland which requires daylight to function and keeps all other hormones in balance. The pineal depends on circadian rhythms to maintain healthy metabolism, happy moods and

2 Hilary Hinton "Zig" Ziglar (November 6, 1926 – November 28, 2012) American author & motivational speaker.
3 http://www.hindawi.com/journals/ije/2010/270832/
4 http://news.uchicago.edu/article/2010/10/03/sleep-loss-limits-fat-loss-study-finds

to activate melatonin production at night. Lack of melatonin, a potent antioxidant hormone that has been shown to protect from cellular ageing, contributes to low moods and diminishes sleep quality. You can increase daylight exposure by using a 'lightbox' in the home, especially in winter months. Lightboxes have been associated with improved wellbeing in the case of seasonally affected disorders (SAD) and mild depression, but they are not a substitute for fresh air and a brisk walk. Avoid using at night.

✓ **Excessive artificial lighting** interferes with the production of melatonin which depends on complete darkness and quality sleep for optimum levels. If you live in a city that never gets completely dark, sleep in total darkness by fitting blackout curtains or blinds. It is important to keep artificial light levels as low as possible at night (especially blue light which has been shown to suppress melatonin), and to avoid exposure to computers, mobile phones and TV screens for at least an hour before sleep. To minimise the impact of your computer at night you can download an app which will automatically cut out the more stimulating blue rays from your screen. Similarly it is possible to buy light bulbs that have had the blue removed and emit a warmer light. Salt lamps are also very good and can be used as bedside table lamps.

Excess artificial light exposure at night and disrupted circadian rhythms (as is the case with night-shift workers) have been shown to directly contribute to altered food eating behaviours leading to obesity[5].

✓ **Lack of movement** or sedentariness has its own metabolism and leads to premature ageing, osteoporosis, muscle wasting and chronic diseases. Movement doesn't just activate muscles, increase blood flow and stimulate metabolism it also ensures that we are interacting with gravity. Without movement and gravity our body will age much more quickly, which is why NASA must find ways to keep its astronauts moving and compensating for the loss of gravity in space. The less we move, the less we want to move and eventually our cells will go on 'stand-by' mode.

A study[6] recently concluded that to be sitting more than three hours a day is associated with an increase of up to 64% in cardiovascular risks even if those people are exercising (30 minutes) daily. This may sound alarmist and I would not want to suggest that heart attack is the destiny of every office worker but if we are regularly sitting at a desk we must also stand up and move frequently (35 times a day is recommended). This will activate our bodies to maintain an 'active' cell physiology, stimulate gravitational interaction, wake up our brains and improve productivity. It is also statistically more beneficial than an average 30-minute workout.

5 http://www.pnas.org/content/107/43/18664.abstract
6 http://www.ncbi.nlm.nih.gov/pmc/articles/PMC3404815/

✓ **High cortisol** levels are associated with depressed immunity, increased blood viscosity, loss of bone density, muscular tension, poor digestion, poor thinking and cellular ageing. It also drives aggressive and compulsive behaviour. It makes us look for ways to suppress discomfort and usually increases cravings for sugar, reliance on drugs and dependence on stimulants and alcohol to get through each day.

The most visible and obvious side-effect of high cortisol levels is of fat deposits around the middle and the upper back – giving that characteristic apple shape and expanding waistline associated with ageing. Generally cortisol levels rise significantly and stay elevated when we are chronically and constantly living from one crisis to another. Too many of us begin the the day sleep-deprived and over-stimulated by caffeine, then rush to work while worrying about a meeting. Never taking time to recover fully from each stress-inducing event is far more detrimental than being confronted with challenges. The former irrevocably drives up cortisol levels, the latter keeps us interested and stimulated. Exercising and sleeping are two of the most powerful ways to recover from stress. Sources of toxicity such as alcohol, sugar and fluoride are other cortisol triggers.

CULTIVATE PERSONAL BEST

There is strength in union but choose your allegiances carefully

We all have our weaknesses. These can be food, behaviour and attitudes that we believe help us deal with the uncertainties and frustrations of life. We defend them because we are attached to their effects or because we believe that letting them go would somehow lead to great suffering. Those attachments are formed in our subconscious through habit, repetition and association. If, as children, we were regularly rewarded for good behaviour with a sweet, it often follows that when we feel neglected and in need of encouragement a chocolate bar or a biscuit can bring this association back. Perhaps smoking is what we did to feel welcome and part of a group (of smokers). It was probably quite difficult at first to overcome the need to cough and feelings of nausea but to be included was a reward worth the effort and we persevered. Years later, a smoker's attachment can be re-enforced again by the desire to belong, but this time to the group that finds giving up smoking difficult.

Groups such as Alcoholic Anonymous and slimming clubs appeal to our basic need to share and feel supported but they fail to recognise that identifying with a 'negatively formulated' objective keeps the group members dependent and attached to their "unhealthy identity". A "negatively formulated" objective is one that focuses on *not* doing something (such as not drinking alcohol) or on a negative behaviour or state required to belong (such as carrying an identifiable amount of excess fat). In 2009 the British government commissioned a study on the shortfalls of their campaign against obesity. Apparently the more we were told that obesity was bad for us the fatter we became. The report concluded that the messages created a category of people called 'obese', which we could easily join by being fat and wishing we weren't, actually made obesity attractive. Not only could we belong, but once we became a member we received special attention, with special policies to help us change and group events to help us feel cared for. That's a strong incentive to stay overweight.

Changing policy by focusing on people who are already incorporating healthy behaviour (while ignoring completely the obese category that made no effort to change) would be the logical conclusion from this report. Surprisingly and despite the problem being correctly identified, the government rebranded its campaign "change4life" and continued to categorise people who were identified solely by their need to change and not by their positive behaviour.

The dependencies and attachments we create are not always healthy and are often anchored in our self-esteem. Recognising our vulnerable self and inherent need for reassurance helps us be creative with our coping strategies when faced with challenges. Most importantly, a particular behaviour is driven, not just by psychological needs, but also by a physiological state. As we commit to improve our health and our awareness, the 'whole' of us changes and the needs and attachments that we have will also evolve to suit the new 'whole' person we have become. No matter how small the steps, the commitment is already changing us.

Recognising individual strength

Our strengths are worth getting acquainted with so that we can use their potential to drive away less desirable elements and accentuate the positive. For example, it is easier to eat more avocados (if you like them) than to eat less bread! Apparently this is all it took, according to a recent survey, for 40% of participants to declare that they were less hungry four hours after their meal if it also contained avocado!. Sometimes it really is that simple.

Keep moving

An activity that you enjoy can be viewed as a way to invest in your health. It is pointless joining a gym if you find exercise boring but if cleaning your house or gardening really turns you on then make that a vigorous and regular activity. It doesn't matter what you do as long as you move your body and you do it frequently and long enough, the benefits to health, longevity, cognitive skills, mood, creativity and self-confidence outweigh every other commitment you can make to your health.

MATCHING GOALS TO YOUR PERSONALITY

We have already seen how a stress response will stem from the unwitting contradictions between what we desire, expect or hope for and our actual life. This section looks at the role personality plays in health and how to understand ourselves better in order to integrate our needs and our goals.

While choice awareness brings the possibility of minimising these contradictions, to understand our own specific personality requirements can help us make choices and adapt strategies that are better suited to us. It also makes us realise that despite what we have in common, everyone is different. Healthy relationships with ourselves and others necessarily means knowing and accepting differences.

SELF-EXPRESSION IS A REFLECTION OF OUR PERSONALITY

While self-expression is important it is only a reflection of how we integrate personality with our values and conditioning.

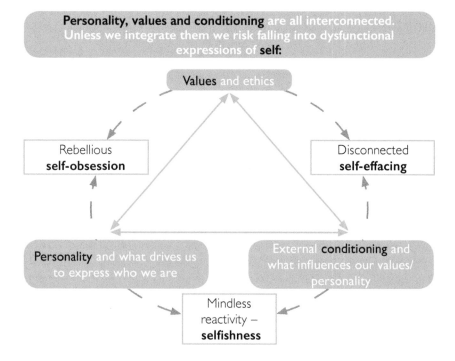

Personality, values and conditioning are all interconnected. Unless we integrate them we risk falling into dysfunctional expressions of **self:**

Values and ethics

Rebellious **self-obsession**

Disconnected **self-effacing**

Personality and what drives us to express who we are

External **conditioning** and what influences our values/ personality

Mindless reactivity — **selfishness**

PERSONALITY NEEDS VS SELF-FULFILMENT

Regardless of our specific personality type, we all share a number of personality requirements. They are the foundations on which we can build a sense of satisfaction with our life. Symptoms of unrest and various degrees of unhappiness usually indicate that one or more of those requirements need to be addressed. They are:

1. Certainty

The need to feel that we are reasonably secure about our future and that our basic needs for food, water and warmth are not immediately threatened. Although we all know that life is unpredictable, we must be able to create a sense of security and certainty about our future in order to thrive.

2. Variety

The need for a certain amount of variety in our daily life to keep us interested and engaged and prevent boredom setting in.

3. Significance

The need to feel that we matter and that we have a place in the world so we can derive meaning for our life.

4. Love connection with others

The need for social interaction.

How we satisfy our basic personality needs is wholly personal but unless we attend to them, we become frustrated. When we are born, those needs don't exist; we are just in a state of being and our parents/guardians are taking care of us. As we grow up, we become aware of the differences between ourselves and our parents. We are our own person and we have to learn who that person is. At first, we do this by becoming conscious of what we are not. Then, as we grow into mature adults we realise our individuality and potential. This process involves the transfer of responsibility for our fulfilment and wellbeing from our parents to ourself. This can be a difficult and painful journey. Personal ownership is not our default setting but it's the only one that will ensure we learn, grow, contribute and thrive. Self-realisation and fulfilment come only once we transcend our personality needs and connect with a higher purpose. Without this essential step we are in danger of only being reactive to our needs without ever finding a purpose. The following diagram illustrates the connections between a higher purpose and self-realisation:

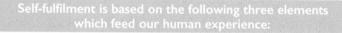

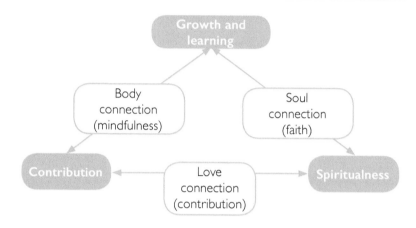

Research has shown that mindfulness[7], gratitude[8] and religious faith are all practices that specifically increase wellbeing, leading to fewer medications and a longer more productive life.

Understanding personality needs and how they can feed into a higher purpose is useful because it makes us ask questions of ourselves and brings awareness about the underlying area a psychological problem can stem from. Indeed events are rarely the cause of trauma, it is our interpretation and our experience of them that causes the unpleasant symptoms. I remember a young girl I once treated who suffered with very severe irritable bowel symptoms. They apparently began after she was raped aged 17 by an older cousin during a family gathering. Initially we discussed the rape, the abuse, the betrayal, the fear, the anger, etc She appeared detached and unemotional. She talked about it describing the emotions that one would expect in such circumstances. I then asked her to tell me about what happened afterwards, not just immediately, but in the months that followed. The question clearly upset her. During that time she was looking for ways to validate her experience and get some perspective on her ordeal. But none came forth. It wasn't a taboo subject: on the contrary it was reduced to a simple rite of passage. Neither her family nor her school friends would acknowledge what had happened as shocking or unacceptable. This not only confused her but made her feel insignificant. Her need for significance was transferred to her bowel which began to play up and make its presence known. Only once she understood this, could she finally move on and find ways to nourish her sense of life-purpose

7 http://www.ncbi.nlm.nih.gov/pubmed/23092711
8 http://www.health.harvard.edu/newsletters/harvard_mental_health_letter/2011/november/in-praise-of-gratitude

YOU'D BETTER
BELIEVE!

More than

2000

studies on the impact of spiritual and religious beliefs on health were published between 2000 and 2009. Most of them show a positive connection between

FAITH AND LONGEVITY.

http://www.tandfonline.com/doi/abs/10.1207/S15327965PLI1303_04#.VeFpw9yrSM8

without the need for severe bowel symptoms. When it comes to our emotional and mental wellbeing it can be useful to ask questions such as:

- Am I feeling angry and frustrated from lack of variety?
- Am I fearful from lack of certainty?
- Am I depressed from lack of connection with others?
- Am I so engrossed in my personality needs that I have disengaged from the overall purpose of my existence?

Each one of the feelings above is connected and interactive. Together they provide a solid foundation on which to welcome fulfilment, be involved in life and source greater vitality.

TO FIND THE EXIT, FOLLOW THE SIGNS

When someone needs an answer from someone who doesn't speak their language very well, they will repeat the question but louder. This is what happens to all of us when our mind can't make sense of something; it just keeps on asking the same question(s) louder and louder. The problem isn't the question, but the way we ask it. If someone has a very limited vocabulary we just have to find a way to make them understand using those words and other means.

The following are examples of useful questions derived from the basic personality needs for certainty, variety, significance and connection with others.

I have applied them to the three main areas of life:

- **Relationships** – with significant other/s but not necessarily a partner
- **Work** – also linked to money
- **Self** – includes our hobbies, creative needs and personal space

✓ **In relation to significant other(s)**

Dysfunctional areas of personality needs	Possible resulting symptoms and feelings	Alternative questions
Certainty/ uncertainty	Anxiety; insecurity; self-doubt; feeling guilty; obsession and compulsion; phobia and fear; depression; substance abuse	Is this relationship a choice? Or am I just afraid of being on my own? Would I feel more secure on my own? Am I being treated with respect? Have I communicated my needs adequately and did the other person show care?
Variety/ sameness	Boredom; habits; lack of sexual interest; numb feelings; unfaithfulness; addictions	Am I involved to fulfil the other's expectations? How do I feel about this person? How am I contributing to the boredom? How can I contribute variety to this relationship?
Significance/ insignificance	Anger; rage; resentment; frustration; depression; regrets	What is my anger/resentment costing me? What benefit do I get from this relationship being what it is? What do I value about this relationship?
Love and social inter-action/dis-connection	Loneliness; rejection; isolation; sulking; aggression; sadness; self-obsession; talkative or silent	What does the other person need? What makes them who they are and motivate their choices? What are they showing me about myself? How can I reach out and contribute?

✓ **In relation to work**

Dysfunctional areas of personality needs	Possible resulting symptoms and feelings	Alternative questions
Certainty/ uncertainty	Anxiety; insecurity; self-doubt; feeling inadequate; obsession; compulsive behaviours; phobia; fear; depression; substance abuse; addictions	Is this position too much responsibility for me? Am I compromising my ethics in this job? Am I chasing the money at my own expense? Is this the only way I can make a living? Can I enlist the support of my family/friends and how will I do it? Can I delegate more? Can I get help and am I willing to ask? Am I simply taking on too much work? How competent am I, really? Have I got a problem with saying No? Am I clear about my boundaries? Am I really that insecure in my work or is it me who is projecting my own insecurities? How can I find out or who can I ask?
Variety/ sameness	Boredom; habitual thoughts; lack of interest; distraction; addiction to violence	How can I challenge myself in this job? What can I do to make it more interesting? What skill would help me improve my work experience? How can I add more variety to this job by contributing to those around me?
Significance/ insignificance	Anger; rage; resentment; frustration; depression; regrets; self-harm	What is my anger/resentment costing me? What benefit do I get from this relationship? What do I value about it?
Love and social interaction/ disconnection	Loneliness; rejection; isolation; sadness; aggression; self-obsession; talkative or silent	Who are my work colleagues? What do my work colleagues need from their work? What are they showing me about myself? How can I reach out and contribute?

✓ **In relation to self**

Dysfunctional areas of personality needs	Possible resulting symptoms and feelings	Alternative questions
Certainty/ uncertainty	Anxiety; insecurity; obsession; compulsive behaviours; phobia; fear; depression; substance abuse; addictions	How can I be more secure in my home? How can I improve my sense of security about my future? What help do I need for this and how can I get it? Is my anxiety rational and what specifically do I dread/ feel insecure about? Can I improve my knowledge about what I am dreading? Am I projecting past traumas into the future? How real/true are my projections about the future?
Variety/ sameness	Boredom; numb feelings; mindless activities, escapism; shopping sprees	When did I last feel excited about something? What made it exciting? How can I creatively reproduce that feeling?
Significance/ insignificance	Anger; rage; resentment; frustration; depression; regrets; self-harm; feeling inadequate	When did I last feel significant and that I mattered? What made it so? How can I make a contribution to my world/ community? What am I saying about myself and how can I improve this in relation to my self-esteem?
Love and social interaction/ disconnection	Loneliness; rejection; isolation; sulking; aggression; sad; self-obsession; talkative or silent; feeling guilty; feeling socially inadequate; shy	When did I last express love and connection to someone? What is stopping me doing this right now? How can I make a positive contribution to my health and the health of others? How can I reach out to others more?

WHICH PERSONALITY?

In psychology, the Big Five personality traits are the five broad domains or dimensions of personality used to describe human personality.

The Big Five personality traits were first used by psychologists to comprehend the relationship between personality and academic behaviours. They have since been used in job interview techniques and to construct marketing and advertising campaigns. The Big Five model is able to account for different traits in personality without overlapping. During studies, those personality traits show consistency in interviews, self-descriptions and observations. Moreover, this five-factor structure seems to be found across a wide range of participants of different ages and of different cultures.

Their relevance here is to better match personality with goal strategies and health behaviour. We all know that if we improved our diet, drank less alcohol, did more exercise and spent more time taking care of our stress levels we would be in better shape. The difficulty may be in obtaining the correct information but after that, we just have to do it (20% aspiration but 80% perspiration!).

The following personality descriptions and recommended associated strategies are loosely based on the Big Five personality traits.

1. **CONSCIENTIOUS**
2. **EXTROVERT**
3. **CONSIDERATE (or AGREEABLE)**
4. **ANXIOUS (or NEUROTIC)**
5. **INTELLECTUAL (or OPEN-MINDED)**

Sometimes it is easier to identify what we are not and what isn't for us. Start by eliminating what doesn't speak to you. After that, take what feels right for you even if it means taking it from more than one personality type.

We can all potentially identify with each of those personality types. Often situations will dictate if we are more conscientious or more anxious. The point of this classification is not to reduce a complex individual to a personality type but to identify a health strategy that will be supportive and useful.

1. CONSCIENTIOUS

Personality description: The *conscientious* person likes to plan, get organised, make lists and pay attention to detail. Changes are prepared meticulously to avoid surprises. Order and rules make them feel secure and unpredictability is unsettling. Fun, rest and play are better enjoyed when earned. A conscientious type requires a minimum of personal space and time to think and de-stress.

- **Strengths:** Action orientated, determined, disciplined, energetic.
- **Weaknesses:** Procrastination, indecision, difficulties prioritising, difficulties adapting to change, likes a routine, critical and easily offended, guilt-complex, self-punishment and inflexibility. Susceptible to stress and can lose focus when routine is disturbed.
- **Helpful strategies:** Writing down objectives with as much detail as possible will help sustain focus even if routine is disturbed. Visualising and spending time daily reconnecting with written objectives will ensure binding commitment. Spending time organising space so that it supports objectives (i.e. the kitchen is adapted to support healthier diet) will make tasks routine. To create pressure and expectation from friends and family by sharing aims and objectives will support their realisation and get past the planning stage. To break goals into small manageable chunks helps to feel rewarded along the way and motivated to continue.
- **Suggested physical activity:** Gym with or without a coach, yoga, hill walking, running, bicycle trips, skiing and swimming. Generally speaking, more solitary activities that can also be meditative.

2. EXTROVERT

Personality description: The *extrovert* needs to feel that they are one among others. Success means lots of friends and a rich social life. Extroverts like to take charge and organise social events. They like to share ideas and tips. Having an audience gives a sense of validation and purpose. Extroverts are action based and usually very energetic.

- **Strengths:** Determined, flexible, adaptable to different situations and people
- **Weaknesses:** Gets easily bored, needs a lot of stimulation and will be easily influenced by contradictory messages or external ideas/input. Loses focus easily and will follow instinct rather than convictions. Does not easily self-motivate. Dependent on appraisal and variety or will give up or become distracted. Can find it difficult to switch off because they thrive on excitement so can also become exhausted.
- **Helpful strategies:** Make a list of the benefits to yourself, not just the goals. Visualise advantages in being healthier and happier in relation to fun and interactions with others. Enlist support and encouragement from friends and family. Better still, get them to join you!
- **Suggested physical activities:** Team games (rugby, football, etc) tennis/badminton/squash, golf club or walking club; any activity done with someone else which forces accountability; sponsored activity for charity.

3. CONSIDERATE (or AGREEABLE)

Personality description: The *considerate* person places people above self. They are emotionally driven and like to feel useful and appreciated. A considerate person can be introverted and very sensitive to others' emotional states and moods. They willingly compromise if it improves a situation or keeps the peace

- **Strengths:** Adaptable and easily satisfied. Holds optimistic views about life and human nature. Tolerant and sensitive of self and others.
- **Weaknesses:** Sensitive to external vibes and internal moods, can lose focus on self. Can get isolated and depressed and not know how to ask for help and support. Assumes that others are needier than self. Asking for support can feel like failure.
- **Helpful strategies:** List the benefits and be accountable to others in getting healthier (i.e. I will be able to help my daughter and my grandson better). Identify an individual with whom to share empathy and goals. Someone who is emotionally close and who will support with kindness. Someone who also needs gentle encouragement.
- **Suggested physical activity:** Group classes (i.e. dance, yoga, Pilates, etc) or one to one coaching. The actual activity is fairly irrelevant as long as it makes it possible to socially interact.

4. ANXIOUS (or NEUROTIC)

Personality description: As the name suggests, the *anxious* person worries. The anxious person easily becomes frustrated and often feels out of control. They tend to react to situations and people and experience life with the sensitivity volume turned up. A negative event can feel as if their whole life is a misery, but something as seemingly insignificant such as a shopping trip can be the most exciting thing ever. The priority of the anxious person is to avoid feeling anxious but in doing so they succeed only in feeling more worried. Situations where they can feel more secure and in control will free their mind and draw on much creativity and inner resources

- **Strengths:** Creative artistic mind. Sensitive and receptive to the environment and the mood of others.
- **Weaknesses:** Easily stressed, gets exhausted and discouraged, rather pessimistic views of the world and fellow man.
- **Helpful strategies:** To find a way to express goals using drawing, brain maps, crafts and by placing certain objects and significant pictures in prominent places. Look to generate positive associations between self and the creative ways in which those goals are expressed. To identify the triggers that cause anxiety is a big step towards self-empowerment and self-control. Seeking

help and support in order to achieve this may be necessary. Consider diet, and food triggers as possible cause of anxiety.

* **Suggested physical activity:** Relaxation, yoga, stretching, walking but also high-intensity exercise like sprinting, spinning, boxing classes, etc

5. INTELLECTUAL (or OPEN-MINDED)

Personality description: The *intellectual* person is always looking for new experiences. They have a vivid imagination and a rich internal life. The Intellectual possesses a sophisticated vocabulary and loves nothing better than formulating ideas and concepts. Learning comes from deep understanding, and convictions become the rules once they have been adopted. The Intellectual is tenacious but can change his/her mind so long as he/she is convinced of the truth of his/her beliefs.

* **Strengths:** Imagination, vivid and powerful mental projections. Committed and likes to succeed.
* **Weaknesses:** Can retreat to mental comfort and disconnect from physical needs. Fantasies and concepts can sometime feel like reality but become a hindrance to achievement. Can be distracted from action. Difficulties making a connection between ideas/concept and self-relevance.
* **Helpful strategies:** Researching and analysing the best method for achieving goals as well as the reasons and health benefits for choosing those goals will make them easier to adopt. Once all this is understood, writing helps to connect with those goals but even better is to say them aloud in front of a mirror or while walking. Also useful is sharing reasons and beliefs about each goal as this will induce a sense of commitment and mental focus.
* **Suggested physical activity:** Responds well to coaching. Activities that have a specific point of focus for centering the mind as well as the body such as golf, target shooting and archery. Martial arts, gymnastics and activities that require mental direction are all suitable.

HOW TO BE OUR BEST ALLY

Everyone agrees that diet and lifestyle have an impact on the outcome of health and ageing, but what of our internal mental chatter that is with us 24/7? Our internal conversation shapes our state of being and therefore influences our diet and lifestyle.

Research has highlighted the potential effects of thoughts on cell conductivity. Certain observable brain pattern activities will be associated with inflammation in remote parts of the body, and hypnotherapy clearly demonstrates that the mind can overcome expected physiological responses, such as pain. To pay attention to what we tell ourselves, and to make the inner voice our best ally is a potentially powerful resource.

However, harnessing the potential power of our internal chatter is not just a matter of replacing negative self-talk with a reframed positive dialogue. Mindlessly telling ourselves that we are wonderful, intelligent and lovable people has no more value than constantly telling ourselves that we are useless. It may be kinder but it is not very effective. A good example is a child who is continuously encouraged to feel it can do no wrong will cease to respond to praise; our mind talk needs to be specific and applied to a specific situation to have positive value. We can justify drinking too much alcohol by either telling ourselves that we are weak willed, or that we deserve it. There is no difference in the outcome; regardless of the positive or negative nature of the mind-talk, we will indulge and possibly go against our best health interests.

FOLLOWING THE BENEFITS

We are all capable of sabotaging our efforts and acting against our best (health) interests and intended goals. In fact Freud went as far as identifying a self-destructive drive *(Thanatos)* which, he theorised, lives in all of us, constantly battling with our more creative life-affirming tendencies *(Eros)*. To recognise that those tendencies exist doesn't necessarily mean that we are simply at their mercy. Whatever drives how we choose to act them out must be linked to the benefits we get from our chosen behaviour. In other words, there are results in both; the life affirming ones and the self-destructive ones.

When a patient, filled with self-loathing, tells me that they feel out of control and wish they were different, I will ask them what benefits they get out of their self-loathing and apparently hateful behaviour. They may find the question challenging but nonetheless relevant. Although we frequently forget, it is an inescapable fact that our free will means we are constantly facing choices which can potentially affect our wellbeing. To identify the benefits of even our apparently most aberrant choices we have to delve into the mind-talk that goes with it.

For instance, in the case of excessive drinking, we might tell ourselves that when joining friends or colleagues in a few glasses of wine it is worth it for the sake of social integration, we don't want to stand out as the "party- pooper", or we may "need" it to suppress anxiety and numb-out feelings of social inadequacy. Sometimes accepting a glass of wine is easier than refusing it; asking for a non-alcoholic drink can turn the spotlight on you, and that might feel worse than the excess weight we would like to lose (even though one drink can lead to another and a hangover can feed self-loathing…).

By looking for the benefits or results in this way we better understand that we feel more socially adequate when under the influence of alcohol, but that opens up the prospect of finding out why we lack confidence when sober. Is it what we tell ourselves? Is it the company that we entertain? Or simply habit? It may turn out that alcohol does very little to enhance our experience other than numb feelings (inadequacy included). By re-evaluating the benefits against the costs, the choice may be less obvious: do we want to feel numb and fat or do we want to feel in control of a difficult situation fully conscious and clear-headed?

The essential, here, is to pay attention to what is going on, add up the benefits, put a value on them, look for an alternative with similar benefits and decide which we would rather choose and why.

Ultimately, when we are choosing there is no right or wrong choice because if we don't like a particular choice we make, we can always change and choose something else next time.

RESISTING CHANGE

Most of the time we are just looking for a way to avoid change…

'Better the devil you know' is our natural default setting. The brain is wired to make certainty where there is none. Our life is potentially totally random. We could at any point trip and fall or collapse and die but we cannot physically maintain that level of vigilance about our life, so we create certainty and probable expectations. That's our survival instinct and the price is a natural resistance to change.

Understandably, when change means losing our sense of security, the incentive is rather limited. When we are looking to change a particular behaviour and we don't succeed, it is frequently because we see it as a dilemma: either I drink, feel socially competent and risk getting fatter or I don't drink and feel socially inept and risk being considered a bore. Whichever way I look at, it I lose. This is also called a double-bind and it means that we are out of choice. To introduce a choice when faced with a dilemma we need to find a third option, an alternative standpoint where we can change without losing and achieve our ultimate goal(s). The followings are three useful ways to get out of a dilemma and move closer to achieving our goals.

1. **Taking an external perspective:** when no matter what I choose, the outcome will be painful or costly, a third option might become clearer by disassociating from the situation. By looking at myself from the outside, I might see that I am neither socially inept nor anti-social, but that the group of people with whom I feel alcohol is needed is the problem and avoiding them is the third option.

2. **Looking for a paradoxical alternative:** My need for alcohol may not be anything to do with an emotional need to cope, but with a physiological need to satisfy the reward pathways in my brain and/or cravings for sugar. What else can I do to satisfy this? How do I ensure that my cravings are better controlled? (the answers to those questions are in the next chapter… read on)

3. **Looking for help:** Instead of cultivating the company of people who always drink in social circumstances I seek the support of someone who understands that I want to stop drinking, and supports my efforts to lose weight and reduce my alcohol consumption.

KEEPING IT STEADY

Lao Tzu tells us that "a journey of a thousand miles starts with the first step". This doesn't just mean that starting is only the most important step; it also means that we have to make each step a goal. So long as we do, we will get closer to our destination. In practice small attainable goals are achievable and anything else is generally a measure of how far we still have to go. Waking up with a hangover and the thought "I will never touch a drop of alcohol AGAIN" is probably as unnecessary as it is unlikely to be fulfilled. On the other hand deciding, *before* meeting friends, that I will stick to a couple of glasses of wine is far more likely to bring success and make me feel that I am in control. Remember: It is far easier to keep balance at a steady pace than to regain control when already falling.

AVOIDING THE ELEPHANT IN THE ROOM

Our consciousness is so wired that it is impossible not to think about something. The minute someone says "don't think of a pink elephant" your imagination will visualise it. The action of not thinking about something is as unlikely as the possibility of a pink elephant walking into the room. Yet we will frequently say to ourselves "I will not do this" or "I will stop eating that". This type of goal is constructed in such a way as to make the task a huge test of willpower at best or even impossible.

Every time we imagine ourselves moving away from something we want to change, we are in fact reinforcing a sense of difficulty and creating failure by strengthening the mental image of what we are trying to avoid. Thus we are creating a vicious circle of avoidance/reinforcement/failure/avoidance. As we say in France: *"plus ça change plus c'est la même chose"* (the more we change the more we keep it the same).

To free ourselves from this self-perpetuating hell, we have to look for an alternative. The desire to stop drinking alcohol becomes the plan to drink sparkling water with a slice of lime. Or, if this is too big a step, to simply limit consumption to one glass of wine with food.

There are alternatives which are much healthier and easy to substitute when cravings hit hard: dark chocolate with very low sugar content makes a satisfying alternative to milk chocolate or a small glass of organic red wine can be a pleasurable contribution to a meal without much damage.

To look for alternatives and be prepared to invest in healthier choices is enough to stimulate an attitude that will power the desired changes. In fact, actively choosing a healthier way of life is the foundation for every goal we may have because it shifts focus from what we don't want to what we do want.

MEASURING ACHIEVEMENTS NOT FAILURE

There is an important, yet subtle, difference between setting goals and the resulting pressure of expectations that ensue. The first is filled with hope and gets us motivated to engage with the task; the latter measures how far we are from our objectives. Excitement quickly gives way to disappointment and a disempowering sense of failure. It is difficult not to be preoccupied by how much further we have to go than by the gains we have already made. Even if the act of measuring achievements is not motivating in itself, we can use those small gains to prevent us from becoming discouraged – and help us to create short term and manageable goals.

MANAGING PLEASURE

Many of us have a confusing attitude towards pleasure. Pleasure is often perceived as 'guilty' and for some the pursuit of it risks turning into an obsession or even addiction. Advertisements for alcohol, cigarettes and online gambling regularly warn us via small print and hidden clauses about indulging 'responsibly' and at our own risk – only adding to the contradictory feelings that we already have about pleasure.

Seeking pleasure is part of our evolutionary hard drive. We have reward pathways in our brain that fuel our desire to reproduce, to improve our existence and to thrive. Evolution closely depends on pleasure because it motivates us to create ways to ensure our safety and our comfort and, ultimately, our survival.

Pleasure is not a measurement of health but it is a consequence of it. It is impossible to sustain a healthy diet and lifestyle unless it gives us pleasure and enjoyment. It's pointless to choose a diet or an exercise programme without first ensuring that we enjoy it. Getting bored with the daily jog or finding a new eating plan dull is the most common reason we fail to keep our New Year resolutions. We are missing out on the greatest motivational power for change because we forget to factor in pleasure!

When setting out health goals apply the following two complementary pleasure principles:

1. **Pleasure is the direct motivation for a choice:** I love a big salad made from fresh crunchy vegetables; I enjoy adding baby leaves and fresh herbs with avocado and roasted pine nuts. Thinking about it makes my mouth water and eating it gives me great pleasure. I like to taste the different flavours, to add spices and delicious exotic oils. To create and reinforce pleasurable sensations around the 'right' choice makes it easier to select.

2. **Pleasure is the reward for our efforts:** I so enjoy the feelings of deep satisfaction and relaxation I get after exercise. My head is clearer, my body feels stronger and my posture is straighter; I feel more confident about myself and more positive about my problems. Thinking about how much pleasure we will derive from our efforts is a very effective motivation for pushing through the inclination to take the easy option.

Pleasure heals and participates in homeostasis or balanced health. Pleasure is not just associated with what we do, eat or drink; we can create it entirely from our imagination. Statistics show that planning a holiday is in fact more beneficial to our health than the actual trip. This is because imagining ourselves having a fantastic time is already stimulating the physiology of pleasure and contributing positively to our wellbeing. In our head nothing goes wrong, the weather is fantastic and everyone is happy – and the advertising brochure confirms it. By simply planning a pleasurable experience, we can trigger the potential health benefits of pleasure "Anytime, any place, anywhere".

Instant gratification is not to be confused with pleasure. It is only a substitute for pleasure. If we are in a hurry or feeling the need for 'a bit of a lift', we will settle for a quick fix such as a chocolate bar or a glass of wine. It gives us some pleasure but it's short lived and it comes with the characteristic rebound sensation that makes us want more and more until we get hardly any pleasure from it, but we have become addicted. What once gave us pleasure, now simply gets us through the day. Addiction is the opposite of pleasure. It is the ghost of pleasure, the gap that's left where there once was pleasure.

Potentially anything that gives us pleasure can become addictive; fortunately not every pleasure comes with harmful side-effects. However, there are some that we need to be wary of. The mother of all addictions is sugar and if combined with fat it is an even stronger trigger, as is the case in junk food (chocolate, hamburgers, bread with lashings of butter and jam, cakes and biscuits). Typically, junk food consumption shares characteristic reward pathways in the brain with addictive substances such as cocaine. For this reason we should be very careful when giving sugar to our children and when eating it ourselves. What makes sugar particularly dangerous and, I believe, the trigger for all other addictions (alcohol, drugs, gambling, sex, etc) is the fact that it is so readily available in concentrated forms. This is complicated by the emotional anchors created from birth. Sugar mixed with fat is in mother's milk and is the first taste babies associate with motherly love. Sugar may be in a large selection of natural foods but it is never isolated. By isolating and then concentrating sugar, food manufacturers have removed the safeguards from the potential ravages of sugar.

If used with discernment, pleasure can be a powerful driving force in our life, but pleasure management must be a conscious activity for us to thrive. Indulging in frequent pleasures that carry maximum health benefits with no undesirable side-effects such as phoning a friend, going for a walk, listening to music or planning a trip to the cinema ensures that our reward pathways are kept satisfied. This protects us from the seductive power of addictive and harmful triggers. However if repeated too frequently, a pleasure can become a habit and lose its rewarding power. To remain pleasurable, an activity must be anticipated and varied.

Pleasure is an expression of happiness and the following is a list of healthy activities that are known to be crucial to happiness, pleasure and longevity.

Expressing gratitude

Psychology has highlighted the many benefits of regularly 'counting our blessings'. It contributes to happiness and helps to put our problems into perspective. To verbally express gratitude to someone is even more potent than simply counting ourselves lucky. In a test participants were asked to read out a letter of thanks to someone they felt especially grateful towards; those who felt the most miserable before expressing gratitude felt the happiest afterwards[9]. Next time you are feeling blue, instead of reaching out for that comfort food, reach out for that special someone and tell them how grateful you feel.

Practising honesty

Research presented at the 2014 national convention of the American Psychological Association suggests that practising honesty by telling fewer lies can significantly improve immune health, self-esteem and happiness[10]. Participants were divided into two groups, a control group and a sincerity group that was told to speak only the truth. Members of the sincerity group were told to speak honestly, truthfully and sincerely – about big things, and about small things, such as why they might be late or unavailable. They could choose not to answer questions but always had to mean what they said.

Lying can come in many guises. Here are five examples to watch out for of how or why we might bend the truth:

1. **Altering or controlling a friend's response** by shading the truth, only telling our side of the story, or altering the way in which we behave to reflect more favourably on us.
2. **Intentionally** leaving out significant/relevant information.
3. **Embellishing** a resumé, exaggerating or diminishing skills, inflating events or changing facts when telling a story.
4. **Downplaying emotions** or pretending not to be interested or involved in order to protect our vulnerable self.
5. **Gossiping** usually involves lying at some point (often by denying the gossip to the person being gossiped about).

Movement

Muscle action directly stimulates brain chemistry. Walking freely and swinging the arms is essential to our brain integration because both hemispheres have to communicate in order to coordinate the right with the left side of our body. This benefits neurological health beyond simple physical activity. Research at Pittsburgh University[11] confirmed that walking substantially protected the brain

---

9 http://www.clidsselfhelp.org/library/counting-your-blessings-how-gratitude-improves-your-health
10 https://cbsphilly.files.wordpress.com/2012/08/kelly-a-life-without-lies.pdf
11 http://www.news.pitt.edu/news/walk-much-university-pittsburgh-study-shows-it-may-protect-your-memory-down-road

from senile degeneration (even if people had already shown signs of dementia) and stimulated the production of dopamine, a chemical critical for coordination, memory function and mood. It is also effective at stimulating creative thought and solutions to problems…unlike alcohol which is a known neurotoxin.

Touch

Touch, like movement, is fundamental to our neurological development and wellbeing. When we are born our nervous system is under-developed and depends on tactile, visual and auditory stimulation to mature fully. Conversely this type of sensation colours our (emotional) feelings. Sensory perceptions are how we know what we feel. As an infant, kinaesthetic perceptions are the first types of sensory perceptions that we experience. Our mother kept us warm, fed, dry and protected from harm by holding, feeding and rocking us. In this way touch became associated with safety and a great source of pleasure. Touch, massage and physical contact can help rectify underdeveloped kinaesthetic perception or simply reconnect us with that powerful feeling of being cared for.

Smell

Unlike other senses, smell is directly connected to the limbic system, the area of the brain involved in adrenaline flow, emotion, behaviour, motivation, pleasure, and even addiction. It has a great deal to do with the formation of memories, which is why smells are often evocative, and our reactions to a smell are rarely neutral – we either like or dislike it. Essential oils can be potent tools to stimulate pleasure (rose, ylang-ylang, jasmine and sandalwood are reputed aphrodisiacs), relaxation (lavender has been shown to induce relaxation) or motivation (rosemary is often used to stimulate thought and intellect). Several studies have also demonstrated that smell can alter social behaviour and make us more receptive to courtship[12].

Music

Music can be a great source of pleasure, and rhythmic sounds are a powerful stimulant to our nervous system. Traditionally music has been used by populations throughout the world to transcend physical planes and access spiritual or altered states of consciousness. In this way it can even be compared to psychotic drugs. Music for many is a true source of joy. It can greatly enhance physical performance and stimulate the desire to move. Together movement and music can transform mood or combine to make us sing.

---

12 http://www.ncbi.nlm.nih.gov/pubmed/11597051

Art and visual aesthetics

Art in its widest forms can stimulate or relax. To pay attention to our environment, and ensure that it is visually pleasing is also a way to bring us into the here and now. Whenever we appreciate a thing of beauty whether a beautiful rose or handmade vase we are forced to bring our attention to that which we admire and centre ourselves in that process. Appreciation (visual or otherwise) is a feeling which has been associated in research with happiness and longevity. Its healing potential has been substantiated by the observation that recalling a time when we felt profound appreciation can improve heart rhythm coherence[13].

Social interaction

Not all social interactions are a source of pleasure, and can sometimes even be quite toxic! But we are social animals and we need to feel that we are part of a community of like-minded people. Feeling isolated is not a pleasurable feeling and there is safety in numbers. By seeking out supportive social interactions we are also stimulating our sense of connectedness and creating higher values. Statistics show that the most common regret expressed by terminally ill patients is that they wished they had made more time for expressing and sharing love with friends and family.

Hobbies

A hobby such as gardening, painting or singing can take us outside of ourselves. The idea is to become so immersed in what we do that we are unaware of the time and in a state similar to meditation. The benefits are very similar but, in many ways, a hobby is more accessible than meditation because it does not challenge us to sit still. A hobby is also a way to connect with our passion and that special feeling of being 'turned on'. Passion, love, enjoyment and getting involved are feelings and attitudes that feed off each other. Passion is contagious and breeds passion but conversely boredom can also numb us to everything and turn off enthusiasm. To make the initial effort to get involved often regenerates a lost passion.

Playing

Playing is a type of interaction and is a social lubricant that gives structure to our relationships by focusing on a shared goal rather than on the individual dynamics. Playing means a game of golf, badminton, football, amateur dramatics, playing cards with friends, singing in a choir or any team building activity that cements interaction with others.

---

13 http://www.heartmath.org/research/science-of-the-heart/introduction.html

LET'S
DANCE!

• •

WAYS TO REDUCE RISK OF DEMENTIA

35%
Reading

47%
Doing crossword
puzzles at least
four days a week

0%
Playing golf

0%
Bicycling &
swimming

76%
DANCING FREQUENTLY

The greatest risk reduction of any activity
studied, cognitive or physical.

From the New England Journal of Medicine

Laughter

Laughter is specific to humans. It can complement social interaction and goes with playing but we can laugh by ourselves. A good comedy film or a compilation of humorous cartoons can do wonders to privately lift a gloomy mood. Laughter activates the diaphragm and abdominal muscles. It neutralises stress, stimulates endorphins and serotonin release, protects the heart and strengthens immunity What's more it activates 15 facial muscles and helps to naturally lift the face, thus improving the appearance of wrinkles!

NATURAL DRUGS

The reward pathways targeted by most anti-depressants can be directly activated by natural substances known to stimulate neurotransmitters such as dopamine and serotonin. They are:

Dark Chocolate

Chocolate stimulates the production of a neurotransmitter (anandamide) that temporarily blocks feelings of pain and depression; it also contains other chemicals that prolong the 'feel-good' aspects of anandamide. Chocolate has even been referred to as 'the new anti-anxiety drug', and a number of studies have confirmed its calming properties. This, of course, refers to chocolate, not sugar which has the opposite effect and no real benefits. Go for high cocoa/low sugar/very dark chocolate and remember that full benefit is obtained by a relatively small dose (35g/day).

Bananas

Bananas contain dopamine, a natural reward chemical that boosts your mood. They're also rich in B vitamins, including vitamin B6, which helps soothe the nervous system, and magnesium, another nutrient associated with positive mood. Just be careful to limit them as they are also a source of sugar.

Coffee

Coffee appears to affect a number of neurotransmitters related to mood control. Research has also shown that coffee triggers a mechanism in the brain that activates brain stem cells to convert into new neurons, thereby improving brain health. Research[14] also suggests that increasing neurogenesis has an anti-depressant effect! Drink coffee without milk for optimum benefit.

Turmeric (Curcumin)

Curcumin is the pigment that gives the spice turmeric its yellow-orange colour. It

---

14 http://www.ncbi.nlm.nih.gov/pmc/articles/PMC2743873/

is thought to be the primary component responsible for many of its medicinal effects (see next chapter for more details). Among them, curcumin has neuro-protective properties that may enhance mood and possibly help with depression[15].

Purple Berries
Anthocyanins are the pigments that give berries like blueberries and blackberries their deep colour. These antioxidants (see next chapter for more details) help the brain produce dopamine, a chemical that is critical for coordination, memory function and mood.

Animal-Based Omega-3 Fats
Found in oily fish (salmon, sardines, mackerel) and krill. One study[16] showed a dramatic 20% reduction in anxiety among medical students taking omega-3. Research has also shown omega-3 fats to work as well as antidepressants in preventing depression.

TURNING ON THE FANTASIES
Imagination is arguably the most powerful characteristic of human intelligence. Imagination makes the seemingly impossible possible. The most unlikely dreams like flying or walking on the moon became a reality because of imagination not just determination. Imagination is a great asset which can be developed and channelled through visualisation, day dreaming and regularly sharing our dreams with others.
I am not suggesting that we disconnect from reality, but consciously projecting ourselves into desirable scenes will stimulate the part of our brain that can and does come up with creative solutions. Seeing ourselves – if only in our imagination – in a successful or happy situation will help us draw on resources to achieve our aims, and will help identify the help we may need along the way.

15 https://pinnaclife.com/sites/default/files/research/Curcumin-Mood-2.pdf
16 http://www.ncbi.nlm.nih.gov/pubmed/21784145

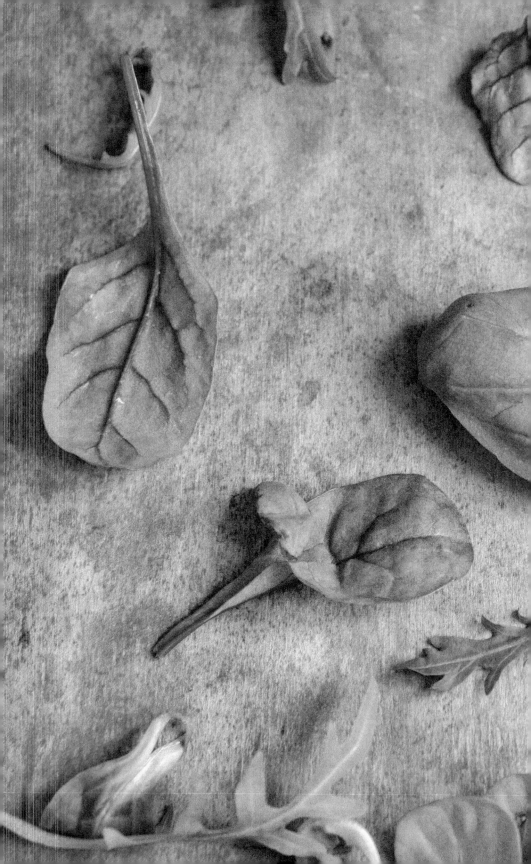

PART THREE:
CREATE HEALTH
FROM WITHIN

*"Stop being a prisoner of your past.
Become the architect of your future."*

ROBIN SHARMA

THE DRIVE TO THRIVE

In this section you'll discover the four essential factors that control health, and how to target the processes that influence ageing both internally and externally.

Our immune system is our ever vigilant bodyguard. At any given moment it is leading a silent and relentless war against a multitude of pathogens and foreign bodies in an effort to preserve the integrity of our tissues.

The digestive system at the heart of our immune system is far more than a tube filled with potent enzymes. It controls everything that penetrates the two-way membrane marking our ultimate boundary. From the food we eat, it filters what can be utilised by our cells for optimum function, energy and repair while simultaneously eliminating unwanted matter and the toxic waste of liver detoxification for safe excretion. Most crucially it is home to the 600 or so strains of bacteria that make up the half of our immune and digestive system that is not human in origin.

Our skin, lungs, liver and kidneys share this crucial function of detoxification thus preventing the multitude of poisons we regularly encounter from causing lasting and irreversible damage. Without these precious organs the coherence of our individual cells would quickly be lost.

Like a brilliant conductor, **our nervous system** coordinates organs and tissues to create harmony from the complicated symphony our biology is playing, while at the same time staying alert and preventing us from walking into danger. The sheer quantity and variety of tasks accomplished by our cells and tissues at any given moment makes the combinations of interactive and influential health factors almost infinite. Good health is a very fragile equilibrium but our bodies are working 24/7 in the most intricate way to keep us alive. All the physiological processes involved in this small miracle are fully interdependent, and the relatively stable equilibrium toward which they aim is called **homeostasis.** By looking at the relationships between our systems and their functions we can begin to create our own good health in a coordinated and connected way. Read on and learn how homeostasis can be supported and how the miracle of your biology can be realised…

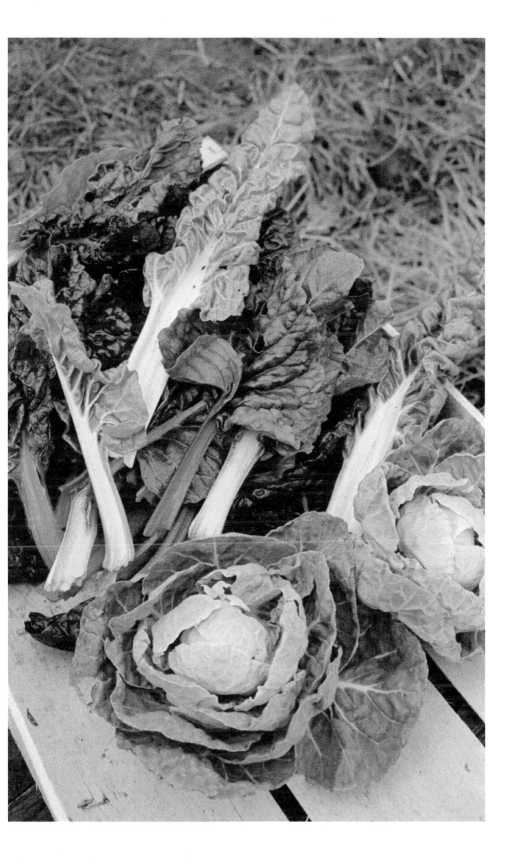

THE SMALL BUT MIGHTY CELL

The cell is the smallest independent unit in our body. Each and every one of our 100 trillion cells, and ten times as many micro-organisms living in and around us, interact to ensure the healthy function of every organ while maintaining the equilibrium of the whole body.

Additionally each cell must preserve its identity and integrity. In our lifetime every cell in our body will renew itself many times over. Who we are today is radically different from who we will be in a year's time, yet we can expect to look more or less the same and for our organs to continue performing through their ongoing turn-over. Ageing is assimilated by the ability of the cells to thrive and perform as individuals, while also keeping to the predetermined fate and tightly regulated role they each must play in the creation of life.

THE FOUR MECHANISMS INVOLVED IN CELLULAR INTEGRITY

They control homeostasis and organ function and can be specifically boosted through diet and lifestyle. They are:

APOPTOSIS (PROGRAMMED CELL DEATH)

Despite continuous cell division, programmed cell death (apoptosis) ensures the number of cells is kept constant in any given organ. This regulatory process maintains the organ's size and shape and is an opportunity to select healthier cells and eliminate individual damaged cells. Apoptosis is an important process in preventing cancer cells from dividing uncontrollably. Selective apoptosis is stimulated by specific fasting methods.

NEUTRALISATION OF FREE RADICALS

Free radicals are positively charged atoms that are mainly the consequence of our oxygen dependence. They are especially damaging to the cell's membrane and DNA. This type of damage is referred to as **oxidative stress**. It contributes to (chronic, low grade) inflammation, cardiovascular damage, skin ageing and organ function failure. The body uses a number of processes to neutralise these damaging free radicals; in particular it recruits electrons from specific **antioxidants** to avoid damage. The majority of antioxidants can be found in the natural pigments that give fruit, vegetables and plants their vibrant colours. Antioxidant status is boosted by eating a wide variety of brightly coloured fruits and vegetables.

SELECTIVE ENERGY SOURCING
Every cell in our body must be able to source energy to function. This is as true of a muscle cell as it is of a brain or a liver cell. The way in which a cell sources energy varies in efficiency. Healthy well differentiated cells are able to obtain energy from both fat and sugar, while deviant unhealthy cells (not well differentiated or cancerous cells) are able to power only on sugar. Cellular adaptability and energetic versatility is a measure of cellular health. The quicker our tissues can go from one type of fuel to another the fitter we feel. Medium chain fatty acids (abundant in coconut fat) and reducing available carbohydrates (especially sugars) from the diet stimulates selective energy sourcing

DETOXIFICATION
Some cells, such as liver and kidney cells, specialise in detoxification, but every cell in our body must efficiently detoxify its own load of poisons. Those are by-products of the cell's function and can also come from its immediate environment. For instance, the cells that line our gut (epithelial cells) will be exposed to the toxins produced by certain gut bacteria, while ovarian cells will be processing high levels of oestrogen. Cell integrity is acutely dependent on the detoxification and elimination of poisons. Reduced glutathione (a peptide made up of the amino acids cysteine, glutamic acid and glycine) is one of the major players in cell detoxification, it effectively handcuffs toxins and escorts them out of the cell for elimination. Glutathione is abundant in whey protein, vegetables, avocados and walnuts, but it is easily destroyed by heat.

THE FOUR ESSENTIAL HEALTH FACTORS THAT CONTROL CELL ENVIRONMENT
The cell's environment is crucial to its functioning because it must ensure adequate supplies of vital elements for energy and repair, while removing the by-products of cellular metabolism and neutralising any toxic or undesirable elements. Those functions are regulated by diet and lifestyle and controlled by the following four essential factors:

I. **Overall toxic burden:** Toxins and poisons are everywhere. We breathe them, drink them, eat them and put them on our skins. They are produced by some of the bacteria that live in our gut and by some of the metabolic processes that take place in our body. The more efficient we are at eliminating toxicity, the less likely it will disrupt cellular integrity. Adequate neutralisation and elimination of toxicity depends on the efficiency of specific organs such as **the colon, the kidneys and liver – and can be stimulated naturally.**

2. **Friendly bacteria and other symbiotic organisms:** Single cell organisms permanently colonise every square centimetre of our skin and mucous membranes. Imagine an army of tiny foot warriors standing shoulder to shoulder protecting a rare and precious army of marksmen trained in chemical warfare (and other weaponry of mass destruction) and made up of our immune cells. This myriad of purposeful organisms is fundamental to our existence and is literally what stands between us and our hostile environment. However, the compatibility between the tissues on which they dwell and the organisms themselves can vary, occasionally producing less than harmonious results. The candida yeasts, for instance, which are responsible for thrush, or specific propioni-bacteria which cause acne, are common examples of disease-causing opportunists while the Bifido-bacteria are some of our more precious allies. By supporting the desirable strains of micro-organisms and discouraging the less welcome ones, we can optimise the health of our immune system and prevent it from using highly toxic warfare. Unfortunately current farming methods, veterinary practices, food processing and the over-prescription of medications from antibiotics to the contraceptive pill have had disastrous effects on our precious bacteria. We are now faced with the consequences of such an indiscriminate approach. **Improving and protecting friendly bacteria colonies will help control the single most persistent cause of premature ageing: inflammation.**

3. **Nutritional status:** Modern agriculture and the over exploitation of arable land has caused the nutritional status of our food to plummet in the last 70 years. It is estimated that the magnesium content of an average cabbage grown in the UK today is half what it was in 1950. Processed food notably brings no nutrition while cooking methods considerably influence the nutritional outcome of our food. Agricultural methods have a significant impact on the nutritional content of food as does storage, preservation and transport procedures. **Without a doubt, food that is grown locally with the minimum amount of pesticides is the most nutritious.**

4. **Overall acid/alkaline balance:** Life as a whole produces acids. Breathing, moving, stress and digestion all create acidic compounds. Specific foods and additives such as salt, sulphur containing proteins, sugar, and additives such as phosphoric acid in cola drinks also contribute to the acidic load. An acid cellular environment has been associated with DNA damage and

with cancers. Acids are especially challenging to the kidneys. The ketone bodies released during fat-burning are also acids and must be neutralised. To effectively neutralise acid compounds we need adequate supplies of organic mineral buffers (sodium, magnesium, potassium and calcium). **The best source is raw vegetable juice which concentrates organic forms of important minerals and makes them the most effective and gentle way to neutralise acids.**

HOW TO TARGET THE FOUR ESSENTIAL FACTORS

An integrated approach to good health is based on the premise that homeostasis is our natural tendency. If we have the knowledge of **how** homeostasis is achieved, we can substantially influence our innate ability to thrive and be healthy. Although this might seem obvious, it's actually the opposite view from the current disease-driven medical perspective! Conventional Western medicine merely exercises damage control and most doctors view health as a slowly deteriorating state all the way to the expected ills of old age.

There are specific measures that support the Four Essential Health factors. I have broken them down into Four Specific Targets and given an outline description for each. How each target relates to your particular state of health is revealed by way of a simple visual questionnaire.

WHERE DO I START?

Health is often the least organised of our priorities. We would rather get the children ready for school, meet a work deadline or fit in a hair appointment than make time to specifically look after our health. To create health and support our natural tendency to thrive we must get involved and be willing to make time for our most precious possession. Prioritising health however doesn't mean to stop enjoying the good things in life or becoming so self-obsessed that we have no time for anything or anyone else. Only by integrating our life with our health requirements can we achieve more permanent health-forming habits that will sustain us fully. As we age, our unique constitution, personality and lifestyle all start to conspire and gradually reveal themselves in specific symptoms. To help you choose which area to focus on I have categorised particular symptoms in relation to the **FOUR** main essential health factors and their targets.

THE FOUR TARGETS OF HEALTH

TARGET 1: TOXICITY

Improve detoxification and reduce toxicity by:
- Recognising and limiting toxicity exposure wherever possible
- Stimulating the detoxification organs (liver and kidneys)
- Increasing output from the elimination organs (skin, bowel, lungs)
- Neutralising toxicity with specific agents like adherents (clays and charcoal) and absorbents (water-soluble fibres)

Turn to page 82 – Detoxification: Why less is more

TARGET 2: CHRONIC INFLAMMATION

Support the immune system and reduce low grade inflammation by:

- Limiting oxidative stress
- Ensuring the diet is rich in antioxidants
- Grounding regularly with barefoot walking (healthy supply of negative ions)
- Reducing dependency on sugar
- Improving essential fatty acid balance
- Preserving gut integrity by reducing the factors that compromise it (gluten, alcohol, chronic and low grade gut infection)
- Limiting allergens (foods and airborne substances that casue allergic reactions)
- Increasing nutrient-dense foods and foods rich in fibre

Turn to page 114 – Inflammation: Putting out the fire

TARGET 3: GUT FLORA

Support digestive health and improve bowel ecology by:

- Supporting the friendly bacteria while staving off the undesirable bacteria
- Supporting and improving digestive enzymes
- Supplementing with fermented foods and specific probiotics (friendly bacteria)

3 **Turn to page 128 – Gut Flora: Making friends of our tiny warriors**

TARGET 4: SUGAR DEPENDENCE

Reduce sugar dependency for energy and get the cell to fuel on fat by:

- Reducing all digestible sugars, grains and starchy foods (potatoes, bread, rice etc)
- Experimenting with food timing to regulate mobilis glycogen (sugar) stores and induce ketosis (the side effect of fat-burning)
- Experimenting with intermittent fasting and juicing days to stimulate and neutralise ketosis
- Exercising and moving regularly
- Addressing stress inducing factors (lack of sleep, lack of confidence, poor relationships)

4 **Turn to page 142 – Sugar Dependence: Burning fat for a change**

HOW TO DESIGN YOUR OWN ANTI-AGEING PLAN (OVERLEAF)

Identify the **symptoms,** follow the **actions** and turn to the **target number**
1 **2** **3** **4** that applies to you:

DESIGN YOUR OWN ANTI-AGEING PLAN

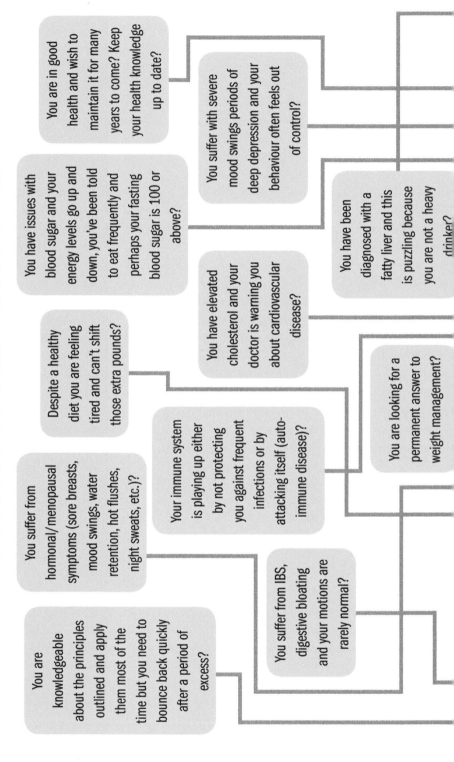

You are in good health and wish to maintain it for many years to come? Keep your health knowledge up to date?

You have issues with blood sugar and your energy levels go up and down, you've been told to eat frequently and perhaps your fasting blood sugar is 100 or above?

You suffer with severe mood swings periods of deep depression and your behaviour often feels out of control?

You have been diagnosed with a fatty liver and this is puzzling because you are not a heavy drinker?

Despite a healthy diet you are feeling tired and can't shift those extra pounds?

You have elevated cholesterol and your doctor is warning you about cardiovascular disease?

You suffer from hormonal/menopausal symptoms (sore breasts, mood swings, water retention, hot flushes, night sweats, etc.)?

Your immune system is playing up either by not protecting you against frequent infections or by attacking itself (auto-immune disease)?

You are looking for a permanent answer to weight management?

You are knowledgeable about the principles outlined and apply them most of the time but you need to bounce back quickly after a period of excess?

You suffer from IBS, digestive bloating and your motions are rarely normal?

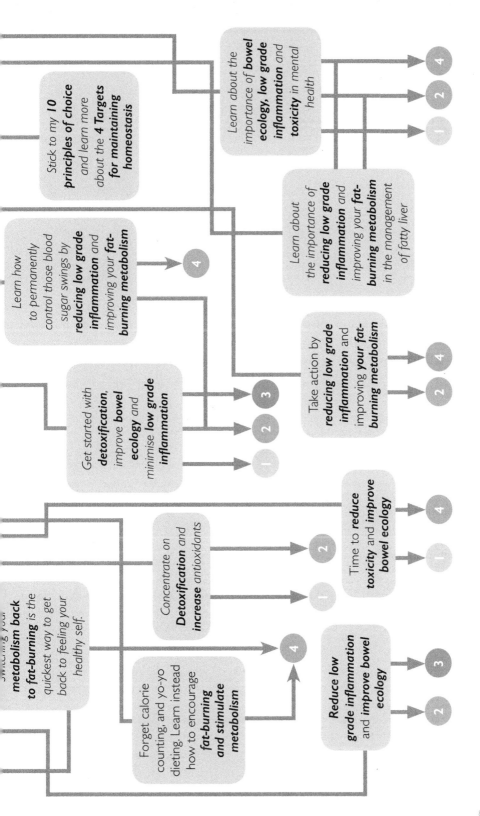

Switching your **metabolism back to fat-burning** is the quickest way to get back to feeling your healthy self.

Forget calorie counting, and yo-yo dieting. Learn instead how to encourage **fat-burning and stimulate metabolism**

Reduce low grade inflammation and improve bowel ecology

Concentrate on **Detoxification and increase antioxidants**

Time to **reduce toxicity** and **improve bowel ecology**

Get started with **detoxification, improve bowel ecology** and minimise **low grade inflammation**

Learn how to permanently control those blood sugar swings by **reducing low grade inflammation** and improving your **fat-burning metabolism**

Take action by **reducing low grade inflammation** and improving **your fat-burning metabolism**

Learn about the importance of **reducing low grade inflammation** and improving your **fat-burning metabolism** in the management of fatty liver

Stick to my **10 principles of choice** and learn more about the **4 Targets for maintaining homeostasis**

Learn about the importance of **bowel ecology, low grade inflammation and toxicity** in mental health

FIRST TARGET: TOXICITY

1

"When I let go of what I am, I become what I might be."
LAO TZU

DETOXIFICATION: WHY LESS IS MORE

Modern life is based on an ever-greater need to consume. Manufacturers are continuously producing new gadgets; agriculture strives to increase productivity at ever-greater environmental costs and the food industry keeps tempting us with new and addictive goodies. Challenging molecules are making their way into our bodies through what we eat, drink, breathe and apply to our skin. Toxic chemicals are deliberately added to our drinking water, supposedly for our own good (fluoride is a typical example). The way in which modern food is processed and packaged has turned it into a health hazard while more recently the seeds themselves are becoming suspicious with dubious genetic modifications. Gases and vapours are belched out by cars, industry, and agricultural spraying. In our very homes lurks danger in the form of toxic perfumes, air fresheners, flame retardants and cleaning products. As if this wasn't enough, poisons can also be synthesised by some of the bacteria in our own gut, depending on the type that colonises it.

Our capacity to adapt is remarkable. In the face of so many new and potentially toxic molecules, our skin, lungs and bowel together with our liver and kidneys still manage to find ways to neutralise and eliminate those poisons. Our ability to detoxify resides essentially with the liver and the kidneys while elimination is with the skin, bowel, bladder and lungs. The thyroid controls metabolic rate which in turn influences detoxification. A fast metabolism means a quick detoxification rate but if some of us can barely handle a glass of wine, while others are drinking like fishes, it is because we are far from equal in our liver detox capacity and our metabolic rate.

Sadly, there are large numbers of poisons to which we are exposed daily that we can't control, but fortunately there are many more that we can avoid by choosing organic foods and toiletries. We can filter our tap water and we can be careful about the type of cleaning agents we use around the home. These measures will go a long way to reduce our toxic exposure. This has been repeatedly confirmed by blood and hair analysis on organic consumers versus non-organic.

GETTING STARTED WITH DETOXIFICATION

Feeling tired, constipated, vulnerable to infections, lacking energy and motivation are all potential signs of toxic build up. Skin texture and colour and the whiteness of the eyes are also good indicators of the need to detox. The first thing people notice when their body becomes cleaner is their skin is softer (especially the rough areas behind the arms, legs and buttocks) and the white of the eyes is clearer. To detox is always a good place to start a health regime or when looking to recover from a serious illness.

TOXICITY: THE ENEMY WITHIN

Our body is continuously metabolising – sorting through food components in order to create new matter and movement. As is the case with **all** energy dependent systems, this process necessitates a proportionate **release of heat** and an efficient **evacuation of by-products**. If the system becomes clogged it will not function efficiently, we'll feel sluggish and vitality will be lost. Our health is a delicate and dynamic balance between input and output. Detoxing favourably influences and maintains that balance.

Just to remind you again, detoxing means to:
Reduce toxicity by recognising and limiting exposure wherever possible
Improve detoxification function by regularly following targeted detox protocols
Stimulate elimination of detox metabolites by increasing output through the bowel, skin and lungs
Neutralise toxicity by choosing specific agents like adherents (clays and charcoal), absorbents (water-soluble fibre) and buffering agents (citrates)

Although it's impossible to completely avoid toxic exposure, we can support the organs of elimination and detoxification.

1 THE COLON: KEEPING THE GATE OPEN

The colon, also called the large intestine, is the last section along the continuous tube from mouth to anus that makes up the digestive tract. The large intestine turns chyme (the liquid left over from digestion) into formed stools as it slowly progresses to the rectum for safe disposal. Strictly speaking the colon is an elimination organ and indirectly supports detoxification. However the bacteria that colonise it have an important capacity to detoxify and digest food residue. The colon is the main gate of elimination for the liver once it has done the job of detoxifying fat-soluble (toxic) compounds.

Our immune system keeps a large portion of its army of reserves (also called Gut Associated Lymphoid Tissue - GALT) along the digestive tract but in particular near the appendix and in the colon. These lymphatic tissues are at the heart of complicated interactions with gut microbes that profoundly influence immunity, inflammation and brain tissue.

To avoid toxic build up, our bowel should easily and satisfyingly open once a day, at the very least. The stools should be plentiful, soft and formed. Variations are perfectly normal but a hard stool, shaped like a small ball signifies constipation. This is usually improved with simple dietary measures but occasionally it can be caused by a low thyroid function, gall-stones or a growth (such as a fibroid or a tumour) obstructing the bowel. Constipation can also manifest as diarrhoea. Bowel symptoms associated with pain, bloating and mucus can be due to Irritable Bowel Syndrome (IBS) and are also the signs of more serious diseases such as Crohn's or coeliac disease. If you develop *unexplained* bowel symptoms, make sure to consult your doctor before attempting any other measures. Bowel function is influenced by many factors, but if you suffer problems with your bowel, I suggest you look at the following:

COLON STRESSORS

Foods that slow down transit and should be reduced:

♦ **Gluten:** as the name suggests, it is a protein that tends to make bowel content more sticky and harder to move. Gluten is a protein found mostly in modern wheat used for making bread and is in a lot of processed foods (pasta, biscuits, cakes, pastries etc). It is often used as an additive to improve consistency. Gluten is also found in wheat, wheat derivatives (spelt etc), rye, and barley.

♦ **Hard cheese and excessive dairy:** Casein in dairy is a protein similar to gluten that can be sticky and binding if consumed excessively, especially when cooked. Casein is most concentrated in hard cheeses.

THE PULSE TEST

Measure your resting heart rate by taking your pulse for 30 seconds while resting in a calm environment. Try taking a few readings to get an average. Normal resting heart rate is between 60 and 80 beats a minute (less for athletes). Faster resting heart rates can be triggered by certain medications, medical conditions and stress/anxiety.

Avoid the food you wish to test for three days prior to the test.

When you eat, your heart rate may increase slightly. Up to six beats above your estimated resting heart rate is normal. However if your pulse goes up more than 12 beats (or beats over 84 beats/minute) after eating a particular food this indicates a possible reaction. That item should be avoided for at least 21 days before reassessing possible symptoms. Take pulse readings at least three times after eating the food over a period of 20 minutes.

Foods that can cause diarrhoea and irritate the bowel:

Any food can cause diarrhoea if it stimulates a reaction from the abundant immune tissue located along the digestive tract. Gut pathogens can combine with specific foods and lead to varying degrees of gut inflammation causing symptoms from colitis and IBS to Crohn's disease.

If a food interacts with the immune system it is either a food sensitivity (delayed reaction) or a food allergy (immediate or short term reaction). Regardless of the speed and specific immune portion, a food should not provoke a defensive reaction. The main consequences of food sensitivities/allergies to the bowel is micro-damage to the intestinal tract lining, contributing to further translocation of toxins from the bowel into the blood and perpetuating a vicious circle of immune reactions and chronic inflammation. This may lead to the sense that you are reacting to most foods when in fact the initial trigger might be to only a few foods.

The obvious foods to start eliminating when experiencing bowel symptoms (IBS, constipation, diarrhoea, flatulence and bloating) are wheat-based foods and dairy products. They are usually processed and overconsumed and contain similar proteins (gluten and casein) which can potentially trigger an immune reaction. The best way to find out if you suspect a particular food is to avoid it for 21 days and assess how you feel. **A pulse test is a quick and inexpensive way to self-test.**

Immune modulated reactions can be measured with various types of testing. Skin scratch test for the antibody most commonly involved in allergy (IgE), blood

THE GUT/BRAIN AXIS

There is a potent neuro-endocrine connection between the brain and the gut which is mediated by the immune system. Studies have demonstrated that under the combined influence of poor diet and gut bacteria, the intestines develop a low grade inflammation. This can lead to a cross-over contamination through the gut brain/barrier to the brain with poisons and toxins leading to behavioural and mental problems. This has been shown to be a contributing factor in Alzheimer's disease*.

The gut is a trove of neurotransmitters (serotonin, GABA and others). Those play an important role in gut motility. They are directly affected by stress and positively contribute to wellbeing. Gut flora has a direct influence on gut serotonin which partially explains why people with disturbed gut flora often report feeling depressed.

The current theory about gut neurotransmitters is that we have developed this sophisticated 'gut feeling' system in order to decentralise awareness and allow the brain to carry out more analytic tasks.

tests for the antibody most commonly involved in sensitivity (IgG) and for other cell related immune factors (such as with the ALCAT test). If a food is shown to activate an immune response it is best avoided until tissue damage is repaired (four to six weeks of strict abstinence) and consumed only occasionally after that (every three to four days maximum).

Factors that impair colon function:

- **Dehydration:** herbal teas and pure filtered water are the best way to keep the bowel hydrated but it also important to eat a diet rich in water dense foods (fruit and vegetables) and water soluble fibres (flax and chia in particular) that have the ability to hold water in the bowel. Ideally you need to drink 1.5 litres of water a day but this varies considerably depending on temperature, exercise, sweating and diet.
- **Ignoring the need to empty your bowel:** this is one of the main causes of constipation and can stem from childhood. Once the habit has set in, it must be rectified with patience and determination. Always go to the bathroom when the urge takes you and start to practise by sitting on the toilet daily at roughly the same time (morning is ideal). Coffee can be helpful and drunk before sitting on the toilet, but any hot drink can be used as positive trigger.
- **Poor positioning on defecating:** in order to empty fully, the bowel must be unrestricted with some assistance from the abdominal wall and diaphragm.

---

*http://www.ncbi.nlm.nih.gov/pmc/articles/PMC3775450/

Sitting is far from ideal for this but squatting is. To simulate squatting while sitting on a modern toilet place a small stool under your feet. Leaning back and forth with your arms above your head also helps with defecation.

♦ **Medications:** there are a number of medicines that can cause constipation, in particular opiates such as codeine, morphine, hydrocodone, oxycodone; antacids; antidepressants; calcium carbonate; ferrous sulphate; and most iron supplements. Be aware of this if you have to take them.

♦ **Excessive methane producing bacteria:** studies have identified a positive correlation between excessive methane production from the fermentation of sugars by certain gut bacteria and constipation. In fact there is also evidence that Irritable Bowel Syndrome and possibly colon cancer are also linked[1]. To control this type of methane-producing bacteria use plenty of oregano and garlic in your food. These herbs have been shown[2] to reduce methane production. They can also be taken in supplement form.

COLON SUPPORT

Foods that encourage a healthy well-functioning colon:

♦ **Fibre, especially water soluble:** linseed, chia seed, psyllium husk, oat bran, whole grains and pulses are the main source of fibre. Fruit and vegetables do contain fibre but less so. To ensure that your diet has sufficient fibre for optimal bowel function I recommend that you include ground flax and soaked chia seeds daily.

♦ **Supplemental gut bacteria:** a very large portion of our stool weight is made up from bacteria rather than food residue. You can improve bowel bacteria status with fermented foods or probiotic supplements.

♦ **Naturally laxative foods:** papaya, prunes, figs, kiwi, rhubarb, Cayenne pepper, (raw) garlic, black pepper, fresh spinach and ginger

♦ **Bowel cleansing foods and their juices:** beetroot, lemon, garlic, cucumber and ginger

♦ **Butyric acid:** a short chain fatty acid produced by Bifido-bacteria in the small intestine from the fermentation of fibre. Butyric acid is also abundant in (organic) butter especially when it is fermented. It is important in maintaining healthy bowel PH and is an anti-inflammatory. It is also available as a supplement.

Bowel cleansing procedures:

♦ **Colonic hydrotherapy:** This is the gentlest method of bowel cleansing. It can be done regularly as part of a bowel training programme and it will positively assist in a juice fast by speeding up the eliminations of the toxins released into the bowel during periods of fasting. Because it thoroughly

1 http://www.ncbi.nlm.nih.gov/pmc/articles/PMC3895606/
2 http://www.ncbi.nlm.nih.gov/pmc/articles/PMC3370521/

cleanses the large bowel it is the ideal opportunity to reseed with desirable bacteria and should always be followed by a course of probiotic (fermented foods and/or supplements). Deep bowel cleansing is useful to manage symptoms of bloating which may develop when adjusting your diet and introducing more vegetables. The effects of colonic hydrotherapy are not just on the bowel. The stimulation of the proprio-receptors in the bowel and the activation of the vagus nerve both encourage gut serotonin (and other neurotransmitters) synthesis. This often makes colonic hydrotherapy an uplifting experience. Colonic hydrotherapy is a great way to connect with the bowel which is an area often steeped in shame and tension. The more relaxed we can feel about our bowel and its function, the better we can trust our gut feeling and create a healthy colon.

- **Enemas:** they can be self-administered in the comfort of your own bathroom. If the idea of lying on the bathroom floor does not appeal or if you are feeling squeamish about sphincter controls try lying in a warm bath when doing an enema. Enemas are a simple procedure to self-manage constipation with the minimum side effects. It is not recommended to do more than two enemas per week for prolonged times as this would disrupt bowel flora. Enemas are also an excellent way to introduce a variety of therapeutic substances. Notably garlic tincture (10ml per 2 litre enema if suffering from parasites or candida and to boost immune system); coffee (use organic freshly ground, simmer 4 tablespoonfuls in 500ml of water, let cool down and top up with cold water) use to stimulate the bowel and liver, especially useful for supporting home detoxes.

- **Herbal laxatives and magnesium salts:** laxatives should not be regarded as bowel cleansers whether natural or otherwise because they will cause irritation and, over time, dependency. However they can sometimes be necessary especially if enemas are not an option. Cascara, triphala or tamarind based compounds are usually gentler than those made from senna or cape aloe. Generally refrain from using laxatives for long periods of time. Magnesium citrate (no more than 2.5 grams per day) can be a gentler option.

2 THE SKIN: OUR BIGGEST ELIMINATION SURFACE

The skin physically stands between us and our environment while allowing exchanges between those two areas. Our skin is highly permeable to fat and water soluble substances and even to gases. Whatever the skin is in contact with, it will be picked up by the myriad of blood vessels that irrigate it and dispatched straight into general circulation. This is unlike the "internal skin" of our digestive tract lining which possesses a parallel blood system (the portal vein) that allows for the blood coming from the gut to be cleansed by the liver before entering general circulation. This makes for a solid argument in favour of cosmetics and toiletries that are as pure and as simple as possible. As with good food, less is definitely more and the quality of the ingredients should speak for themselves without needing adjusting and masking. If after checking the ingredients in your facial cream or body lotion you are baffled by the chemistry and not tempted to taste it, I suggest that you change it.

The skin is also a fantastic elimination organ that can excrete quantities of toxic compounds through the sweat glands. It's important to keep the skin free from the dead skin cells that are continuously shed through its surface by regular and gentle scrubbing and/or by dry skin brushing. However make sure to keep your brush (or scrubbing gloves) impeccably clean by regularly spraying them with colloidal silver (from health stores) or hydrogen peroxide (from chemists). Anti-perspirants are an aberration since they block this major elimination function and should be avoided. They also have been associated with increased breast cancer in younger women[3] and contain toxic chemicals best avoided.

SKIN STRESSORS

Toxic substances to look out for in cosmetics and toiletries:

- **Parabens:** widely used preservatives to prevent the growth of bacteria, mould and yeast. Parabens possess oestrogen-mimicking properties associated with increased risk of breast cancer. These chemicals are absorbed through the skin and have been identified in breast biopsy samples. They can be found in body-lotions, make-up, body washes, deodorants, shampoos and facial cleansers. You can also find them in food and pharmaceutical products.

- **Synthetic colours:** those are labelled as FD&C or D&C, F represents food and D&C represents drug and cosmetics. These letters precede a colour and number (e.g., D&C Red 27 or FD&C blue 1). They are coal-tar and petroleum derived, both are suspected carcinogenic and skin irritants and are linked to attention deficit hyperactivity disorder (ADHD).

- **Fragrance:** a meaningless term created to protect a product's "secret formula" but without much regulation. Often associated with allergies, dermatitis, respiratory distress and potential effects on the reproductive system. 'Fragrance' is found in many products such as perfume, cologne, conditioner, shampoo, body wash and moisturisers. Perfumes and fragrance are highly volatile compounds easily absorbed by the skin and lungs. Use essential oils such as lavender or fragrance free products, instead.

---

3 http://www.ncbi.nlm.nih.gov/pubmed/21337589

TO USE SUNSCREEN OR NOT TO USE SUNSCREEN?

The ingredients in sunscreens are often toxic. To limit this, look for an organic product and accept the fact that the ingredients will make it rather thick and sticky.

Ultimately the problem with sunscreens is that they tend to limit vitamin D synthesis and lull us into a false sense of security, so we end up staying in hot sun far too long. Even if the skin doesn't burn, over exposure can still cause sun damage. The more tanned the skin is, the more resistant it is and the recommendation is to gradually build a tan with sun exposure no longer than 20 to 30 minutes at the beginning and never more than 90 minutes. Reserve sunscreen for the more delicate and exposed parts such as your face hands, arms and the top of your feet and shoulders.

- **Phthalates:** a group of chemicals used in hundreds of products to increase the flexibility and softness of plastics. The main ones used in cosmetics and personal care products are dibutyl phthalate in nail polish, diethyl phthalate in perfumes and lotions, and dimethyl phthalate in hair spray. They are known to be endocrine disruptors and have been linked to increased risk of breast cancer, early breast development in girls, and reproductive birth defects in males and females. Unfortunately, they are not disclosed on every product when added to fragrances (often the 'secret formula' not listed). This is a major loophole in the law. They can be found in deodorants, perfumes/colognes, hair sprays and moisturisers and sex toys.

- **Triclosan:** is a widely used anti-microbial chemical, a known endocrine disruptor (especially thyroid and reproductive hormones) and a skin irritant. Triclosan has been shown to contribute to the development of antibiotic-resistant bacteria. Triclosan can be found in toothpastes, antibacterial soaps and deodorants. Ordinary soap and water is enough to wash off pathogens from the skin and there is no evidence of additional benefit from using antibacterial soap.

- **Sodium laureth sulfate (SLS)/Sodium lauryl ether sulfate (SLES):** This surfactant can be found in more than 90% of personal care and cleaning products (think foaming products). SLS is known to be a skin, lung, and eye irritant. A major concern about SLS is its potential to interact and combine with other chemicals to form nitrosamines, (a carcinogenic molecule associated with ageing). These combinations can lead to other issues from kidney damage to lung irritation. They can be found in shampoo, body wash, mascara and acne treatment.

- **Formaldehyde and formaldehyde-releasing preservatives (FRPs):** are used in many cosmetic products to help prevent bacterial growth. This chemical was deemed a human carcinogen by the International Agency for Research on Carcinogens (IARC) and vapours have been linked to cancers of nose and throat. It is known to cause allergic skin reactions and it may also be harmful to the immune system. It can be found in nail polish, nail treatments, bodywashes, conditioners, shampoos, make-up cleansers and eye shadows.

- **Toluene:** a petrochemical derived solvent listed as benzene, toluol, phenylmethane or methylbenzene. It can affect respiration, cause nausea and irritate the skin. Toluene has also been linked to immune system toxicity and birth defects. It can be found in nail polish, nail treatments and hair colour/bleaching products.

- **Propylene glycol:** an organic alcohol commonly used as a skin-conditioning agent. It's classified as a skin irritant and penetrator. It has been associated with causing dermatitis as well as hives in humans even at very low dilution. It can be found in moisturisers, sunscreen, make-up products, conditioners, shampoo and hair sprays.

- **Sunscreen chemicals:** they function as a sunscreen agent, to absorb ultraviolet light. These chemicals are endocrine disruptors and are believed to be easily absorbed into the body where they create cell damage and disrupt DNA. Common names are benzophenone, PABA, avobenzone, homosalate and ethoxycinnmate. They can be found in sunscreen products and other lotions.

- **Aluminium and aluminium salts (alum):** the main ingredient/s in deodorants and antiperspirants – even those which claim to be natural. Aluminium has been shown to be absorbed through the skin and is a neurotoxin connected to neuro-degenerative diseases.

- **Per-fluorinated compounds – also known as a PFC:** they are fluorinated chemicals used extensively for their non-stick slippery properties as surface coating in Teflon and stain/water repellent textiles. More to the point they can be found on dental floss. PFC are carcinogenic compounds known to disrupt immune, liver, and endocrine systems. More worryingly still they are almost impossible to break down and detoxify and will gradually accumulate in the body. Choose a specified wax coated dental floss and avoid non-stick cookware, and stain repellent fabrics/carpets.

SKIN SUPPORT

Skin detoxing measures:

◆ **Saunas:** (hot or infra-red) and steam rooms all promote sweating and encourage detoxification of the lymph, and tissues. Raising body heat also helps kill viruses and bacteria and saunas/sweat lodges can benefit the immune system considerably. To be most beneficial you will need to go back into the sauna at least three times with periods of rest in between to encourage further sweating. You can also frequently rinse (no soap) with cold water to encourage circulation. Aim to stay in the sauna as long as is tolerable and necessary to induce profuse sweating.

◆ **Skincare:** The skin is protected by colonies of friendly bacteria. These must also be cared for in order to keep the skin healthy and resistant to infections (fungal and bacterial). Excessive washing, especially with antibacterial soap and shampoo, is damaging to those delicate organisms as are skin PH variations. A skin PH above 6 starts to affect skin flora and from 7.5 upward will strip them radically. Most tap water value is 8 or more and soapy water will shoot up to 12. To best care for your skin protective flora, prepare a 25% dilution of apple cider vinegar in a spray bottle mixed with your favourite smelling herbal tea and/or floral water. Apply it on your hair and body after (or instead) of washing. You can also add lemon juice or apple cider vinegar to your liquid soap or shampoo to positively influence its PH. Look for very simple soaps such as "soap nuts" (the soapy element comes straight from a plant and requires no additives), Castile soap or Marseille soap. Aim to have as few different skin care products as possible. Oils such as Argan oil, and butters, such as cocoa and shea, make wonderful moisturisers, cleansers and facial creams while pure floral waters make perfect toners and cleansers.

3 THE LUNGS: HOW GASES ARE DETOXIFIED

The lungs are the site of gaseous exchanges between the oxygen that is necessary for cell respiration and carbon dioxide which is released after combustion of the main cellular energy sources (sugar, amino acids and fatty acids). Lung function is regulated by carbon dioxide (CO_2) concentration and not by the need for oxygen (O_2), although one is a consequence of the other. The more critical is CO_2 because it acidifies the blood and this is life threatening. In practical terms this means that in order to maintain a healthy blood pH we have to remember to breathe out. Most of us, especially under the influence of stress and habit, will either hyperventilate or take in too much air by mouth breathing. The advice to take deep breaths when stressed would be more useful if specifically applied to exhaling.

LUNG SUPPORT

To encourage healthy breathing:

- **Conscious breathing:** Regularly focus on your breath. Aim to make it slow and quiet. Count two to inhale and four to exhale
- **Abdominal breathing:** Most people use only their chest and shoulders when breathing. To help shift the breath from the narrow part at the top of your lungs to the wider part at the bottom, you must engage the diaphragm. Practise diaphragmatic breathing by placing one hand on the chest and the other on your belly below your rib cage; breathe deeply and slowly; ensure the chest is staying still and only the belly is moving.
- **Deep postural and core muscles exercise:** Posture affects our ability to breathe freely and effectively. Improve your posture by making sure you keep your back straight and by strengthening the muscles in your mid-back with rowing movements. Engage your core muscles by keeping your balance while standing on one leg then the other.
- **Nose breathing:** Most people open their mouth when they breathe or when they start to increase movement but this is not necessary. Close your mouth and practise nose breathing when moving and exercising. If you sleep with your mouth open (this is often associated with back sleepers and snorers), train yourself to nose breathe while sleeping. You can buy special adhesive chin strips to help keep your mouth closed. Nose breathing is an important step to alkalise the body and control low grade inflammation.

4 THE KIDNEYS: DETOXING AND FILTERING THE BLOOD AND REGULATING ACID ALKALINE BALANCE

The kidneys filter the blood. They process our five litres of blood up to 25 times a day and eliminate urea, a by-product of protein breakdown from old cells, immune activity and diet. The kidneys detoxify water soluble compounds and regulate water balance to maintain steady blood volume regardless of variations in hydration. The kidneys control blood composition, notably mineral salt concentration (i.e. sodium, potassium, and calcium), tissue pH, and blood pressure. They also regulate calcium absorption through the activation of vitamin D, and excrete the end-products of filtration and detoxification via the bladder and urine. The kidneys play a critical role in maintaining blood pH, regardless of variations in food, respiratory rate and movement intensity. However this is at the cost of mineral buffers such as magnesium, potassium and calcium citrates and to the detriment of cellular pH. Over time an acidic cellular environment reduces cellular health and has been associated with inflammation and cancer[4].

Excess amount of sodium chloride (table salt): Refined salt in particular is acid forming and a stress to the kidneys.

4 http://www.cancerci.com/content/13/1/89

SODIUM CHLORIDE AND HIGH BLOOD PRESSURE

Sodium chloride is a denatured and refined form of table salt. It is used extensively in processed foods as a taste enhancer and a way to mask otherwise bland foods. It is a very cheap preservative. The more salt in a food the better it will keep. It is found excessively in baked goods (breads, biscuits, Danish pastries.) and cheeses, as well as the more obvious crisps, popcorn, bacon and processed meats.

It has an acidifying effect on the body, and the kidneys have to work extra hard to neutralise it. This is the most likely mechanism by which sodium chloride (table salt) has been found to contribute to high blood pressure.

However, salt should not be vilified indiscriminately. Natural salts, such as Atlantic sea salt or Himalayan (pink) salt, contain far less sodium chloride (no more than 87%) and come with their own package of up to 86 alkalising trace elements. Furthermore sodium chloride is essential to health and when used sparingly for taste enhancement has no negative effects on blood pressure or heart health.

KIDNEY STRESSORS

Common substances to avoid:

- **Nitrate and nitrite:** Found in water supplies affected by agricultural spraying (farm workers are especially vulnerable), nitrate and nitrite toxicity comes from their propensity to bind to amino acids and create carcinogenic compounds (NOC) – especially damaging to the kidneys and colon. They are also used as preservatives in industrially cooked/processed meat such as ham, turkey and sausage, listed on packaging under codes E249 and E252. They can be present in meat and milk in varying concentrations, depending on how the animal is reared. Intensive farming substantially increases nitrate/nitrite levels in those products so aim to consume organic meat and dairy whenever possible.
- **Alcohol:** A poison that has to be metabolised in the liver, alcohol disrupts electrolyte balance (sodium, potassium, phosphorus and magnesium) in the kidneys. It directly contributes to water retention and (uric) acid build up and is a major cause of joint inflammation and kidney stones.
- **Phosphoric Acid:** Found in carbonated drinks, this inorganic and corrosive

acid works well for descaling the kettle but is a major stressor to the kidneys' delicate buffering system. A study[5] demonstrated that those who drank as little as two colas per day were at increased risk of kidney disease. The more they drank the greater the risk regardless of the type (diet or regular) and the brand of cola. Phosphoric acid is such a strong acid that in order to neutralise it the kidneys will resort to taking calcium from the bones leading to kidney stones and osteoporosis[6]. Although it is found in most sodas, it is much higher in cola flavoured drinks

- **Sugar:** We increase blood sugar levels and cause broad spectrum tissue damage whenever we eat sugar (see section on inflammation for more details). The kidneys are particularly susceptible to this and kidney failure incidence is much greater amongst diabetics. This is regardless of insulin use which provides no significant protection against tissue damage from raised blood sugar as stated in a number of studies published in the New England Journal of medicine between 2008 and 2009. Sugar is also a heavy contributor to the acid load on the kidneys, further depleting their precious buffers. When our kidneys find themselves short of buffers they search for alternatives and end up using those stored in our bones and muscles (rather than in our precious organs and brain). There is also growing evidence of increased uric acid levels from sugar consumption. Raised uric acid levels are directly connected to elevated blood pressure, kidney stones and joint pain.

Other substances to watch out for:
- **Excess sulphur-containing amino acids (cysteine and methionine):** are acid forming and therefore a stress to the kidneys' buffering system. For this reason excess protein from a high meat diet can lead to osteoporosis, kidney stones and uric acid build-up. Sulphur-containing amino acids are essential to health (unlike processed foods and drinks). Excess animal protein is a problem only if we fail to also consume abundant alkalising vegetables and fresh fruits alongside. Protein requirements vary depending on gender, age and activity levels. As a general guide aim to eat no more than 110 g of meat or fish per meal and never more than once a day.
- **Excess calcium:** Together with the parathyroid, the kidneys regulate the concentration of calcium in the body. When we consume excess calcium it is expelled in the urine, and depending on the type of calcium it may precipitate and lead to kidney stones. This is particularly true of calcium carbonate used in processed foods, some medications (antacids) and cheap calcium supplements (frequently prescribed for osteoporosis). Calcium

5 http://www.ncbi.nlm.nih.gov/pubmed/17525693
6 http://www.ncbi.nlm.nih.gov/pubmed/17023723

CALCIUM SUPPLEMENTS AND OSTEOPOROSIS

Calcium carbonate is the most common prescription for osteoporosis – yet it is poorly absorbed. Osteoporosis is a far more complex condition than a simple deficiency in calcium. A recent meta-analysis* concluded that calcium carbonate contributes to kidney stones and bone spurs and, even more concerning, could cause hardening of arteries. The acid form of calcium and magnesium (citrate or malate) is far better absorbed and less likely to cause problems. Far more effective in the prevention of osteoporosis is to make sure your diet is rich in alkalising vegetables; magnesium (found in seaweeds, green vegetables and almonds); and vitamin K2 (found in natto, a kind of fermented soya 'cheese'). Some cheeses (brie and gouda, in particular), will also support calcium absorption in the bones.

According to Professor L. Kervran, (French scientist, born 1901), the body has the enzymatic capacity to manufacture calcium and magnesium from silica. This is how chickens make egg shells and cows produce so much calcium-rich milk from grass. Cucumber, tomatoes and cold-pressed cacao are rich sources of silica which has also been shown to contribute to strong hair and nails and to prevent skin losing its elasticity.

Weight bearing exercises are fundamental to osteoporosis management. Squatting, with weights if possible, has been shown to trigger the Human Growth Hormone (HGH) involved in the synthesis of new bone and muscle cells. Vitamin D is also vital for healthy bones.

must be in correct proportion compared to magnesium. This is difficult because frequently our diet contains too much calcium from calcium enriched foods (cereals, soya milk, etc) and dairy products and not enough magnesium. Magnesium regulates important physiological functions from energy creation to smooth muscle relaxation (heart, blood vessels, bowel and organs). Magnesium has been shown to benefit blood pressure and help prevent sudden cardiac arrest, heart attack, and stroke. It is necessary for teeth and bone formation and nourishes the nervous system. To optimise magnesium levels consume plenty of organic green leafy vegetables, nuts and seeds. Foods with high magnesium content include seaweed, coriander, pumpkin seeds, unsweetened cocoa powder, and almonds.

♦ **Heavy metals:** are pervasive in our environment and a common source of toxicity in the body. Because of their ability to reabsorb and accumulate divalent metals (an atomic property shared by a number of metals including

*http://www.ncbi.nlm.nih.gov/pubmed/21505219

the toxic/heavy type), the kidneys are the first target organ of heavy metal toxicity. Heavy metals are associated with a multitude of slow developing chronic diseases from Alzheimer's to MS and from cardiovascular to auto-immune diseases. Our ability to detoxify heavy metals is influenced by many factors from gut bacteria to genetic factors. Because of this some of us will have a propensity to accumulate heavy metals, especially in the heart, kidneys, thyroid and brain tissues, where they will cause chronic disruption and eventually disease. Heavy metals are detoxified through the liver and kidneys and eliminated through the bowel, urine and sweat. It is possible to measure heavy metal toxicity levels through a specific hair analysis.

The most common and toxic heavy metals we are exposed to:
Aluminium: is the most abundant metal in the Earth's crust. It is naturally absorbed from the soil by plants and foodstuffs. While 50 years ago we may have ingested minute amounts from vegetables (and possibly from some of the pots in which they were cooked), today it is found in almost everything. Aluminium salt has properties that make it a versatile and useful additive. It can be added to water for improved clarity and to foods that contain raising agents such as breads, cakes and biscuits because of its excellent anti-caking properties. It also enhances colouring and can be added to sweets, fizzy drinks and most processed foods. It is naturally found in tea, cacao and wines, depending on regions and growing methods. Its optical property makes it an ingredient of choice in cosmetics and sunscreens; it is the main active ingredient in antiperspirants and deodorants (even the 'natural' crystal deodorants).
As a buffering agent aluminium can be used in medications like aspirin, antacids and vaccines and for improved consistency in talcum powder and toothpaste. We know aluminium can be toxic, yet there is no legislation to govern its concentration in anything other than in drinking water. Additionally aluminium can migrate to food from cookware and packaging materials such as foil and cans. As much as 20% of aluminium in the diet may come from packaging, according to the US Food Standards Agency.
Cadmium: is highly toxic and a component of the metallurgical industry, battery manufacturing, certain paint pigments, phosphate fertiliser and cigarette smoke. Air and water contamination is more common near industrial areas but cadmium has been found in paint used on cheap jewellery, toys and knick-knacks produced without strict manufacturing standards. It is also found in poorly farmed shellfish (check the provenance and go for organic!).
Mercury: is toxic to the nervous system and is used in certain fungicides, algaecides and insecticides. This has contributed to the contamination of some food products,

REMOVING MERCURY FILLINGS SAFELY

You will find different protocols and approaches to removing mercury fillings. Choosing a dentist who is aware of the danger of mercury to you (and to the dentist) is preferable to releasing quantities of mercury dust and vapour in your nose, mouth and the environment (a leading cause of water pollution). For a list of mercury aware dentists in the UK you can visit: www.mercuryfreedentistry.org.uk

Mercury fillings don't behave in the same way with everybody – effects vary depending on saliva pH, bacteria colonisation in the mouth and diet. I strongly recommend that if you have a number of 'silver' fillings or metal caps hiding mercury fillings and you are susceptible to infections, and/or suffer with osteoporosis, mental health issues, Alzheimer's, MS, ME, arthritis, Grave's, Crohn's, allergies, or any auto-immune disease, that you consider removing the mercury from your mouth.

For one month prior to the first dental appointment, throughout the period of removal and for a further two months after completing removal I recommend that you take twice daily:

- 3g combination of soluble fibre (ie. psyllium husk and apple pectin)
- 1.5g activated charcoal
- 1.5g N-acetyl cysteine
- 5g spirulina or broken cell walls chlorella
- A strong antioxidant combination containing vitamin C

During that time, be sure to incorporate regular detox days (see menu planners in Part 5)

particularly grains and cereals. It can also be released from burning (news)papers that have been treated with mercury containing fungicides. It negatively affects zinc and selenium levels in the body and is often implicated in low thyroid function. Sulphur containing foods such as garlic prevent its absorption from food. Mercury is found in 'silver' amalgam fillings. Those should be carefully avoided, especially because of their proximity to the brain. If you already have amalgam fillings it may be wise to think about replacing them but you must be careful to remove them safely.

Another major cause of mercury toxicity is from industrial coal burning. This is the main reason why oceans are now contaminated and large fish-eating fish (tuna, shark, king mackerel, swordfish, halibut, etc) are frequently found to contain relatively high levels of mercury. Smaller fish (sardines, mackerel etc), shrimps, scallops and organic farmed fish are generally found to contain low levels of mercury.

Lead: is found in cigarette smoke, old paint, old pottery (avoid for eating or drinking), and if your drinking water still goes through old fashioned lead pipes. Petrol used to contain lead and largely contributed to the current level of environmental pollution. Until recently this kind of fuel was still allowed for air traffic and agricultural purposes. A complete stop on lead in gasoline was finally imposed by the United Nations in 2013. Lead displaces calcium and is deposited in joints thus contributing to arthritis.

KIDNEY SUPPORT

Pure Water: it is very difficult to know what is in our drinking water, so I recommend the use of a water filter as a way to control quality. Bottled spring water can be very rich in nitrates. Additionally, there is the inherent problem associated with plastic bottles which are known to leach BPA (bisphenol-A). Several different quality water filters are available; look for a reverse osmosis filter or one that can remove heavy metals, hormones and pesticides as well as chlorine. Our hydration needs vary considerably depending on diet, climate and sweating. It is difficult to establish the ideal amount of water you should be drinking but very often thirst is mistaken for hunger and it is good practice to have frequent sips of water. Keep a glass by your bedside, desk and drink while exercising.

- **Naturally diuretic foods:** parsley, watercress, beetroot, black radish, chervil, asparagus and celery; add them to your fresh juices and foods.
- **Organic potassium:** is a potent buffer that supports kidney function and maintains good acid-alkaline balance. Organic (i.e. from a living source) potassium is not the potassium chloride found in salt substitute. It is found in avocados, in most vegetables especially celery, beetroot, asparagus, apricots and in many fruits as well as in coconut water.
- **Lemon and citric acid:** not to be confused with ascorbic acid (vitamin C) is an organic acid and a natural component of many (citrus) fruits. It inhibits kidney stone formation. Unlike calcium, potassium, or magnesium citrates, which are often prescribed to alkalise the urine, citric acid does not alkalinise the urine but rather prevents small stones from becoming "problem stones". It does this by coating them and preventing other material (including bacteria), from attaching and building onto them. Lemon

juice is the richest source of citric acid. It can be used as a natural flavour enhancer and preservative in juices, salad dressings and water.

◆ **Herbal support:** Dandelion leaves and flowers, blackcurrant leaves, raspberry leaves, ginger, uva ursi, barberry, birch bark, gravel root, golden rod and juniper berries can be used in cooking, tinctures and herbal teas

◆ **Saunas:** The composition of sweat and urine are closely related. The skin is often referred to as the 'third kidney'. Use saunas to encourage elimination of many water soluble poisons through the skin and take the burden away from the kidneys.

3 THE LIVER: OUR INTERNAL CHEMIST

The liver is a major detoxification organ. It turns large, toxic and insoluble compounds into small and soluble elements that can easily find their way for elimination through the kidneys, sweat glands and bile system.

The sheer load of potential poisons and toxins that our liver has to deal with is phenomenal. Each and **every second 310kg of toxic chemicals are released** into our air, land and water by industry around the world. This amounts to approximately **10 million tons** of toxic chemicals released into our environment each year. Of these, over **2 million tons** are **recognised carcinogens**. This amounts to about **65kg** each second and there is nothing we can do about it!

In order to cope with even the most complicated molecules the liver has a two-step system of chemical processing. Phase one utilises a sophisticated panel of detoxification enzymes to prepare each molecule for the neutralising action of phase two. The compounds that come out of phase one are highly reactive and potentially even more damaging than their parent molecules. Phase two is critical to detoxification because it has to match the speed at which phase one releases reactive and toxic molecules.

If the liver becomes congested with excess fat, slows down under stress or lacks vital nutrients (especially B vitamins and amino acids) we risk auto-toxicity. The typical symptoms are fatigue, brain fog, headaches, muscle pain, chronic inflammation and neurological symptoms such as anxiety, restlessness, irritability and depression. All such symptoms are associated with toxic burden and can be improved with supportive liver detoxification. They are also frequently associated with 'detox reaction'. A more accurate description of those unpleasant side-effects would be a 'retox' reaction. Too many toxins are pushed out of our fatty tissues into general circulation where they can create havoc if the liver is not fully able to cope. Although this is sometimes unavoidable, by increasing elimination through the bowel, kidneys and sweat glands while supporting liver detoxification, it is possible to minimise the symptoms of auto-toxicity.

FRUCTOSE METABOLISM AND FATTY LIVER

Fructose is the main type of sugar found in the high fructose corn syrup used in processed foods and drinks. It's also in foods aimed at diabetics, honey, dates, maple syrup and agave syrup. Regular white/brown sugar (from cane or beet) is also 50% fructose and 50% glucose. Fructose is the main sugar in fruit, but because fresh fruit is also very rich in water and fibres the fructose concentration is reduced. However fruit juices and dried fruit will considerably *concentrate* the fructose content.

Fructose has a very different metabolism from glucose. Unlike glucose it does not raise blood sugar because it is taken straight to the liver via the portal vein system thus by-passing general circulation. However once it gets to the liver its metabolism follows virtually the same pathway as alcohol and creates very similar havoc when in excess. In particular it leads to visceral adiposity (belly fat), fatty liver (non-alcohol induced cirrhosis) and increased uric acid level. Fructose is a major stress to the kidneys and a known cause of elevated blood pressure and joint pain.

The liver can comfortably metabolise about 25 grams of fructose per day. This should be reserved for fruit and will be quickly reached if you eat three pieces of fruit per day. A medium orange contains about 6 grams.

The bile system is another detoxification pathway (especially for hormones). It emulsifies fats and is involved in fat digestion. Dietary fats stimulate bile release from the liver into the duodenum where it stimulates digestive enzyme production, regulates gut pH, gut motility (peristalsis) and bowel ecology.
If we minimise additional stress from foods, beverages and habits and support our liver's detoxification process., it will reward us many times over. The liver has an awesome capacity to accommodate and is the organ that regulates digestion and energy distribution as well as detoxification.

LIVER STRESSORS

Food and drink damaging to the liver

◆ **Alcohol** must be detoxified by the liver. This process releases an intermediary molecule, acetaldehyde, which must be neutralised rapidly to avoid surrounding tissue damage. This process uses up the potent antioxidant Glutathione. Glutathione reserves are in limited supplies. Additionally acetaldehyde requires a specific liver enzyme to break down (acetaldehyde dehydrogenase) which can be in short supply in some people and explain variations in tolerance, but regardless of this alcohol is a liver stressor and acetaldehyde a known carcinogenic. Additionally alcohol is metabolised straight into liver fat.

- **Fructose,** unlike glucose, does not get used up as energy but is converted straight into fat. This process can only take place in the liver and contributes to the intra-abdominal fatty deposits associated with obesity and metabolic syndrome.
- **Lactose** found in dairy, is made up of one molecule of glucose and one molecule of galactose. Galactose has an identical metabolic pathway to fructose and if eaten in excess will contribute to fatty liver. If you have issues with (non-alcoholic) fatty liver then avoid all milk-based dairy products.
- **Trans fats** result from heating unstable and unsaturated vegetable oils. They are also used by the processed food industry because they are cheap and have excellent shelf life. Despite tighter regulations on the use of trans fats, they are still found in margarine, fake butters and fried vegetable oil. How a vegetable oil is extracted also accounts for trans-fat content. All industrially produced vegetable oils like corn, peanut and rape oils are heated when extracted thus producing a non-negligible amount of trans fats.

Habits and substances that challenge liver detoxification:
- **Rapid weight loss** tends to store toxic molecules in the fatty tissues out of the way. Rapid weight-loss will free those poisons at an alarming rate and stress the liver. There is evidence that the benefits usually associated with lower body weight are negated when weight-loss is too quick. This is not a reason to give up on the whole idea of reducing body fat, but it does confirm that yo-yo dieting actually contributes to ageing.
- **Low-fat diets** are damaging to the liver because they limit bile output from the liver and contribute to gall stones and bile congestion. The liver needs fat to stimulate bile which is a major route of detoxification. Low fat diets are also damaging to hormonal balance and health as a whole.
- **Large meals consumed late at night.** At night the liver is involved with detoxification rather than digestion, and should not be processing large amounts of rich foods.
- **Too frequent eating.** Because the liver has a dual function of digestion and detoxification it needs periods away from digestion in order to attend fully to detoxification. In fact a period of fasting is regarded as one of the best ways to let the liver concentrate on and maximise its detox ability.
- **Smoking and recreational drugs:** all release poisons that stress the liver
- **Toxic products applied to the skin and in your environment:** be mindful

of cosmetics, toothpaste, cleaning products, washing powders, perfumes, paints, air fresheners etc

* **Medications:** Be mindful to take only what you have to without exceeding the prescribed dose. Ibuprofen overdose leads to serious liver damage. Just because something is sold over the counter does not make it harmless.

LIVER SUPPORT

* **Lecithin** is extracted from soya or sunflower and occasionally egg yolks. and is a rich source of phospholipids (notably phosphatidylcholine) which is an abundant constituent of cell membrane and an essential bile precursor. Choline has been shown to be supportive in the treatment of fatty liver and cirrhosis and is a precursor to the neurotransmitter acetylcholine involved in many neurological functions particularly muscle contractions and memory. Choline is a very potent antioxidant (methyl donor) that supports liver detoxification. Phospholipids help keep cholesterol (a major constituent of bile) more fluid thus preventing gall stones forming and the liver becoming sluggish. Lecithin also encourages fat-burning metabolism and is a useful adjunct to detoxing. It comes in granules or capsule forms; make sure to source a non genetically modified lecithin.
* **Healthy fats:** are found in wild or organic oily fish, pasture-raised or wild meat, egg yolks, avocado, un-roasted nuts and seeds (including coconut), flax and hemp oil
* **Coffee:** A number of studies and meta-analysis (6) have correlated coffee with reduced risk of liver cancer. It seems to inhibit gene expression for inflammation especially in the liver.
* Antioxidants in coffee, such as chlorogenic acid, have also been shown to improve glucose metabolism and insulin sensitivity. Drink your coffee filtered and black. Choose organic coffee as it is a heavily sprayed crop otherwise.
* **Foods and herbs that are bitter and encourage bile flow:** chicory, endive, radicchio, artichoke, dandelion leaves and roots, gentian, burdock, camomile
* **Liver tonic herbs, foods, and juices:** beetroot, radishes, daikon, black radish, carrots, onion, garlic, cabbage, broccoli, kale, rosemary, peppermint, horseradish, turmeric, saffron, lemon, ginger, Cayenne pepper, milk thistle.

THE DETOX PLANS

Whichever detox you choose, remember that your body has to be in a relaxed state otherwise it is not a detox but an additional stress. During your detox be particularly gentle with yourself for the maximum benefit.

Expect to feel more tired and do not be alarmed if your sleep is disrupted, you get a headache or feel nauseous. Those are all temporary symptoms related to the process. Make sure to drink plenty of fluids and to rest.

BOOSTING YOUR DETOX

To encourage relaxation, make sure that you get plenty of quality sleep, go to bed early, use blackout curtains and avoid stimulating bright lights.

Equally important is what you choose to read, watch on television and listen to. When we are relaxed our subconscious is especially receptive to the information that is coming our way via radio, TV and newspapers. Listening to the news or watching violence has a significant impact on health and wellbeing. People who involve themselves in world news on a daily basis have been shown to be significantly more depressed than their less news-conscious counterparts. This is thought to be due to the overwhelming feeling of helplessness in the face of so much wrong in the world.

Three active principles that can boost your detox:

1. **Reducing digestive demand** and freeing energy for detoxification. Digestion takes up a lot of energy and the organs involved in digestion (liver, bowel and pancreas) are also involved in detoxification. The less we ask them to digest, the more they can detox.

2. **Reducing calorie intake** and forcing the body into using up old cells, freeing toxins from fat cells and sourcing energy from damaged or unhealthy tissues. Research has now demonstrated how the body operates a careful and selective priority system when in a state of reduced energy supply by burning what it does not need and preserving vital and healthy tissues and organs.

3. **Stimulating the organs of detoxification and elimination with specific detox-boosting protocols.**

Things to consider before you begin a cleansing programme:
*   Do not undertake any kind of detox if you are ill without medical consent and the supervision of a practitioner.
*   If you are on medication or on the pill there is a strong chance that the medication/pill will be flushed out of your system more quickly than usual while you are on a detox. Avoid unprotected sex and check with your doctor with regard to your medication(s).
*   If you have an eating disorder I recommend that you get the support of a professional practitioner and the consent of your counsellor before doing a detox.
*   If you are already underweight I recommend that you address all the other aspects described in this book before considering a detox and seek professional advice at the same time.

FUNCTIONAL STRESS AND SIRTUIN: THE SECRET BEHIND DETOX DIETS

Sirtuins are a group of proteins at the forefront of current research on anti-ageing. They are implicated in a wide range of age-related cellular processes from genetic transcription and mitochondria biogenesis (creation) to apoptosis and inflammation.

Humans possess seven sirtuins that can be found within the cell's compartments; namely the nucleus (genetic material), the mitochondria (energy production) and the cytoplasm (cellular matrix). Sirtuin activity is a function of age. It specifically regulates energy and alertness and is stimulated by intense physical activity (exercise) and calorie restriction (a characteristic of any detox diet). Sirtuins make the difference between good and bad stress and the reason why detox diets are such powerful anti-ageing interventions.

Resveratrol (a polyphenol/antioxidant) has also been shown to increase sirtuin activity (SIRT 1 specifically controls ageing genes) and makes a powerful argument in favour of small amounts of red wine and very dark chocolate. However, as part of a detox it's best to favour dark berries, dark grapes, turmeric, green tea, parsley and kale as they are excellent sources of resveratrol without the inconvenience of added alcohol or sugar.

THE THREE-DAY LIVER DETOX

The objective of the cleanse is to stimulate the liver to excrete bile, to support detoxification with specific herbs and foods and to minimise toxic stress and digestive requirements.

Liver Detox Tea:
10g gentian roots
10g dandelion roots
10g rosemary leaves
20g liquorice roots
1 ltr water
Directions: Simmer and drink through the day.

Dead Sea Salt Bath (or Epsom salts):
Use 300g per bath. Make it as hot as you can bear for at least 20 minutes before going to bed. This is a great way to get both magnesium and sulphur into the body and support liver detox.

Choose if you suffer with a lot of digestive bloating, burping, acidity and/or if you know that your liver is showing signs of stress (fatty liver, elevated ALT enzymes, gall stones, etc) but check with your doctor if you have a medical condition. This cleanse is also great for clearing emotional blockages as the liver is traditionally associated with frustration, resentment, feeling stuck and anger.

It is fundamental to good hormonal balance and I have found that this cleanse will help with rectifying most hormone-induced symptoms like hot flushes, PMT, vaginal dryness, breast symptoms and metallic taste in the mouth. Right shoulder pain with no known reason and which does not improve with bodywork also frequently improves with detoxing the liver. I recommend that you repeat this cleanse every three to four weeks until symptoms disappear and thereafter four times a year to maintain the benefits.

You can easily combine this cleanse with a liver and gall bladder flush on the second day.

DETAILS:

- Limit food intake to **ONE green smoothie** and **TWO vegetable juices** (favour broccoli, peppermint, beetroot, lemon, carrots, ginger and turmeric)
- Drink **ONE** litre of the Liver Detox Tea each day
- Take 5ml standardised organic liquid extract of Milk Thistle **THREE** times daily

TIME	TIMETABLE
On waking	5ml standardised organic liquid extract of Milk Thistle
9:00	300ml juice – any combination of vegetables recommended for Liver Detox. (see Detox Recipes) Add 1 level tsp of spirulina powder and 1 level tsp of lecithin granules
12:00	5ml standardised organic liquid extract of Milk Thistle
14:00	300ml juice – any combination of vegetables recommended for Liver Detox. (see Detox Recipes) Add 1 level tsp of spirulina powder and 1 level tsp of lecithin granules
16:00	5ml standardised organic liquid extract of Milk Thistle
18:00	Green Smoothie. (see Basic Recipes) Add 1 level tbsp of organic whey protein concentrate 1 level tsp of spirulina powder and 1 level tsp of lecithin granules
Before bed	Bath with Dead Sea salts

THE LIVER AND GALLBLADDER FLUSH

This is done over a minimum period of two days but you can include it in any cleanse or detox. It forces the liver and gall bladder to excrete a large amount of bile by challenging it with (olive) oil on an empty stomach. Bile is one of the routes of excretion of toxins from the liver through the bowel. Bile expression is the result of the liver contracting and the greater the amount of oil, the stronger (and therefore more uncomfortable) the contraction and release of bile. To complete this process it is necessary to wash the bowel with a strong laxative or a colonic hydrotherapy treatment otherwise the bile, and the toxins it contains, risk being re-absorbed. Bile pellets that contribute to liver congestion will also be expelled in this way thus preventing the formation of gall stones. If you have liver or gall bladder disease seek medical advice before doing this cleanse.

THE NIACIN FAT-BURNING SAUNA METHOD

You will need to buy niacin (a type of vitamin B3 which induces a strong flushing reaction). Look for 100mg tablets. Take 50mg of niacin per 20kg of body weight; wait 20 minutes, then exercise for 20 minutes to break a sweat and stimulate circulation. Follow up with a hot sauna. You can come out regularly to cool off under cold water and to drink before going back in. Stay as long as you can, up to one hour. The niacin will make you flush and sweat and will induce slight itchiness/tingling. This is normal. It will also stimulate fat and cholesterol breakdown which is where the body stores a lot of very toxic chemicals like DDT.

You can finish off by taking either five activated charcoal tablets, or some clay, which will bind with toxins, allowing them to be eliminated through your GI tract. Just make sure you do not take it in combination with medications or supplements, as these will also be bound up and eliminated.

This method has been shown to help process and eliminate a variety of toxic chemicals and has been used successfully with the firefighters involved in the 9/11 disaster[*]. Use to complement any detox or on its own.

---

[*]http://www.lewrockwell.com/2014/05/joseph-mercola/detox-made-easy/

TIME	TIMETABLE
Night before flush	Stop eating at 6pm
On waking	Only consume vegetable juices and/or fresh raw vegetables and fruits until 2pm.
14:00	Dissolve 2 round dessertspoonfuls of Epsom salts (from thechemist) in cold water and add the juice of a lemon. Prepare this ahead of time to ensure that the salts are properly dissolved. Keep refrigerated.
17:00	Take half the Epsom salts and lemon juice mixture. Expect that the Epsom salts will give you diarrhoea after 30 minutes to 3 hours depending on your bowel.
19:00	Take the second half of the Epsom salts and lemon juice mixture. **Do not drink any more fluid (except olive oil and grapefruit juice below) until the next morning.**
22:30	Mix the juice of a pink grapefruit with 120ml (160ml for larger people) of olive oil in a screw top jar and shake vigorously. Drink the mixture and go to bed. Prop yourself up on pillows and avoid lying flat for the first hour or if you are feeling nauseous during the night.
Following morning	Take a further two doses of Epsom salts or have a colonic hydrotherapy treatment (colonic irrigation or home enema). It's important to rehydrate the day after the flush. Some people experience nausea or may even vomit, however these are symptoms that will improve as your liver becomes stronger from doing this flush. You can repeat it every 4 to 8 weeks.

THE FIVE-DAY KIDNEY CLEANSE

The objective of the cleanse is to stimulate the kidneys, reduce acid build-up and dissolve kidney stones.

Kidney Detox Tea:
20g dandelion leaves
20g golden rod powder,
20g meadow sweet
1.5ltr filtered water
Directions: Simmer gently for 10 minutes. Strain and drink the tea throughout the day.

Sauna:
Aim to do at least three saunas during the cleanse. Make sure to keep well hydrated. For more information on saunas see info box.

This cleanse is useful to alkalise tissues and address issues relating to the kidneys and bladder such as bladder infection and kidney stones. It is also a great way to reduce water retention and improve the appearance of cellulite. Emotionally, the kidneys relate to fear and indecision. Cleansing the kidneys will help you to move forward in life with confidence and greater creativity. Use it to ease joint pain and arthritic conditions. It can be repeated every six weeks providing that it does not aggravate your symptoms. If this is the case I recommend that you look at starting slowly with the more general recommendations before embarking on the Five-Day Kidney Cleanse.

DETAILS:
- Limit food intake to **THREE** Kidney Detox Juices made with any combination of celery, cucumber, beetroot, parsley, coriander, chervil, fennel, ginger and turmeric root
- Add the juice of citrus fruit (lemon, orange, grapefruit) but no more than two fruits per juice
- Drink **1.5 litres** of the **Kidney Detox Tea** each day
- Take **one** level dessertspoon of **marshmallow** root powder in hot water **THREE** times daily

TIME	TIMETABLE
On waking	I dessertspoon of marshmallow root powder in hot water with the juice of ½ a lemon Stevia root can be used to sweeten
9:00	300ml Kidney Detox Juice – any combination of vegetables and fruit recommended for kidney detox (see Detox Recipes) *Must include the juice of at least one lemon or lime but no more than two citrus fruits *Add ¼ tsp (1500mg) of kelp powder
12:00	I dessertspoon of marshmallow root powder in hot water with the juice of ½ a lemon Stevia root can be used to sweeten
14:00	300ml Kidney Detox Juice – any combination of vegetables and fruit recommended for kidney detox. (see Detox Recipes) *Must include the juice of at least one lemon or lime but no more than two citrus fruits *Add ¼ tsp (1500mg) of kelp powder
16:00	I dessertspoon of marshmallow root powder in hot water with the juice of ½ a lemon Stevia root can be used to sweeten
18:00	300ml Kidney Detox Juice – any combination of vegetables and fruit recommended for kidney detox. (see Detox Recipes) *Must include the juice of at least one lemon or lime but no more than two citrus fruits *Add ¼ tsp (1500mg) of kelp powder
Before bed	Unlimited Bone Broth consommé (see Basic Recipes) If you are vegetarian replace this with potassium broth consommé (see Basic Recipes)

THE SEVEN-DAY BOWEL AND TISSUE CLEANSE

The objective of the cleanse is to alkalise the tissues in order to help detoxify the cells while stimulating elimination through the bowel.

This is a longer cleanse which focuses on the bowel. It is done in combination with daily enema or colonic hydrotherapy and will cleanse all tissues. It is great to detox heavy metals or chemicals that you may have been exposed to. It will improve constipation and aid weight loss. It can be done two or three times a year to boost the immune system and ensure that your body is staying healthy and strong. A great way to reset the body after periods of stress. Although I recommend this cleanse for seven days, it can be done for periods of between three and 21 days depending on what you want to achieve. However, I do not recommend it for longer than 21 days without taking a break of a minimum of three weeks regardless of your condition and the reason for doing it. To take breaks from it will make it far more effective than doing it for long periods of time. It is also deficient in essential fatty acids and amino acids.

DETAILS:

This is a juice-based detox that incorporates probiotics with psyllium husk, apple pectin, charcoal and clay. Together they have the ability to absorb and bind to the detox metabolites (the compounds left over after detoxification) that the body dumps into the bowel in order to shuttle them out for their safe elimination. They also reduce potential toxic load from bowel bacteria.

Twice daily enema: To stimulate bowel release you can add green coffee to your morning enema and camomile tea to your evening enema. Home enema kits are available online.

However, **colonic hydrotherapy** is far more effective than an enema. If you can get to a practitioner then aim to include at least **THREE** colonics per **SEVEN-DAY TISSUE CLEANSE**.

TIME	TIMETABLE
On waking	Mix by stirring: I tbsp of psyllium husk I tsp of clay (green or bentonite) I tsp of apple pectin ½ tsp of activated charcoal Add water and continue stirring. Drink quickly
10:00	300-450ml of fresh juice of your choice with limited fruits (see Detox Recipes for ideas) *Add I tsp of spirulina and I tsp of lecithin *Take I capsule of a strong probiotic
12:00	Mix by stirring: I tbsp of psyllium husk I tsp of clay (green or bentonite) I tsp of apple pectin ½ tsp of activated charcoal Add water and continue stirring. Drink quickly
14:00	300-450ml of fresh juice of your choice with limited fruits (see Detox Recipes for ideas) *Add I tsp of spirulina and I tsp of lecithin *Take I capsule of a strong probiotic
16:00	Mix by stirring: I tbsp of psyllium husk I tsp of clay (green or bentonite) I tsp of apple pectin ½ a tsp of activated charcoal Add water and continue stirring. Drink quickly
18:00	300-450ml of fresh juice of your choice with limited fruits (see Detox Recipes for ideas) *Add I tsp of spirulina and I tsp of lecithin *Take I capsule of a strong probiotic
Before bed	Unlimited Bone Broth consommé (see Basic Recipes) If you are vegetarian replace this with potassium broth consommé (see BasicRecipes)

SECOND TARGET: CHRONIC INFLAMMATION

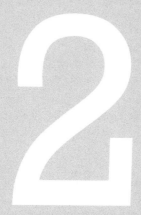

*"Victorious warriors win first and then go to war,
while defeated warriors go to war first and then seek to win."*
SUN TZU

INFLAMMATION: PUTTING OUT THE FIRE

We all experience acute inflammation when we cut ourselves and for a while the area around the cut is red, swollen and sore. As the tissues reform, the inflammation ensures that potential invaders are kept at bay and dead tissues dealt with until the cut has healed and inflammation is no longer needed.
Inflammation is a highly effective response from the immune system to deal with tissue damage and support repair. Inflammation relies on potent chemicals (including destructive free radicals) to neutralise and digest invaders such as viruses, bacteria, yeast or damaged tissue from cellular activity or injury.

IMMUNE RESPONSE: AN EFFORT IN DAMAGE LIMITATION

As with any chemical warfare, inflammation is a non-specific response and for that reason comes with collateral damage of surrounding tissues. It works well in a crisis (a viral attack or physical trauma) but can become chronic and overly destructive when dealing with something which is an ongoing feature such as grass pollens or an internal trigger from gut bacteria, a dietary protein or a cellular process. While external and foreign invaders stimulate **acute** inflammation, fatty acid balance (from food and adipose tissues) significantly controls **chronic** inflammation. One of the mechanisms thought to induce chronic inflammation is the regular bursting of fat cells as they become engorged. This is a common problem associated with obesity and insulin resistance. The immune system will mistakenly start to treat those damaged fat cells as foreign and set in motion a process of chronic inflammation. Chronic inflammation is now well documented in the formation of arterial plaque and the progression of diseases such as dementia/Alzheimer's, MS, diabetes, allergies and all auto-immune diseases. Because of its aggressive nature, it is a major contributing factor to ageing. By reducing chronic inflammation we can positively influence degenerative diseases, slow down ageing considerably and address some of the factors underlying auto-immune symptoms.

FREE RADICALS: SURVIVAL IN THE LINE OF FIRE

Oxygen-dependent cellular activities such as movement and energy production rely on the transfer of electrically charged ions. This creates instability (free radicals) within the cell, which makes it vulnerable to the ravages of oxidation. The cellular structures that are particularly sensitive to oxidation are the cell's membrane and DNA (especially mitochondrial DNA). Electron-hungry free radicals are also created by the sun's radiation and through air pollution, smoke, food, drinks, etc.

To protect the cells from excessive oxidation, we need an ample supply of negative ions from dedicated molecules that can easily sacrifice themselves to oxygen without becoming unstable themselves. These are the precious antioxidants, which are plentiful in colourful plant leaves, fruits and flowers, where they protect the plant from excessive sun damage while still being able to use sunlight as a source of energy.

OXIDATIVE STRESS AND CHRONIC INFLAMMATION: CONTROLLING THE ENEMY

Oxidative stress has been the subject of much research because it combines with, and is created by, chronic inflammation. Together they are directly implicated in ageing, tissue hardening, skin wrinkling and cancer.

Oxidative stress is the inspiration behind claims that cosmetics may slow down ageing when enriched with antioxidants such as vitamin A or coQ10. Howeve, the theory that all antioxidants are created equal and for the purpose of automatically neutralising free radicals is not supported by research. Indeed vitamin E and beta-carotene supplements have been shown to aggravate smokers' risks[1] of developing lung cancer under certain circumstances. Those studies do not show that antioxidants are damaging to health but that, as with everything else in biology, we need to look at the whole interaction rather than oversimplify causes and effects. When eating a food that contains a package of complementary antioxidants that includes vitamin E and beta-carotene (eg in organic apricot) we are consuming numerous synergic molecules together with the life force that informed it into a coherent whole. This is obviously far more harmonious to our own health than isolating a singular molecule and synthesising a lookalike from inorganic materials in a laboratory.

As with all complex biological expression, chronic inflammation is multi-factorial. It can be controlled by reducing the contributing causes within the body, in its environment and at the interface of the two – namely the gut wall.

TO CONTROL LOW-GRADE INFLAMMATION AND OXIDATIVE STRESS:

- Ensure your diet is rich in antioxidants
- Ground regularly with barefoot walking
- Reduce sugar dependency and processed foods
- Avoid burnt foods
- Improve essential fatty acid balance
- Preserve gut integrity by reducing gluten, alcohol and processed foods
- Limit allergens (foods and airborne substances that cause known reactions)
- Increase nutrient-dense foods

GROUNDING AND HARVESTING NEGATIVE IONS FROM EARTH AND WATER

20 minutes of regular barefoot walking on damp earth (such as a dew-infused lawn) or damp sand is a simple and effective way to harvest precious, antioxidant negative ions. Also useful is breathing sea air because the constant stirring of water creates negative ions. The work of Dr James Oschman on the benefits of harvesting negative ions (also called earthing) shows promising results. It is particularly useful in the management of inflammation and pain.

If you don't have regular access to the sea or damp earth, you can buy earthing shoes, mats and sheets.

EXTERNAL AND DIETARY FACTORS THAT DIRECTLY CONTRIBUTE TO CHRONIC INFLAMMATION

I. Airborne allergens (pollen, dust mites, moulds etc)

They are common and can be reduced by regular vacuuming, good ventilation and anti-dust mite measures. Use wool bedding as dust mites do not thrive in wool. Wool is also naturally non-flammable and does not require spraying with nasty flame retardants. Organic washable cotton, bamboo, wool and silk are considered the least allergenic fabrics for clothes and underwear. Ultimately allergies improve considerably with appropriate nutrition because the health of the immune system is closely dependent on food and digestive health.

2. Trans fats

Despite tighter regulations imposed by Europe on trans fats we are far from protected from the harmful effects of processed vegetable oils. Vegetable oils are mass produced and extracted under considerable pressure and heat from corn, soya, canola and rapeseed. This process damages the fragile fatty acids and creates toxic pro-inflammatory fats, which are found in ordinary vegetable oils, dressings, ready meals and whenever vegetable oil is mentioned on a label. Even more toxic and severely inflammatory are the aldehyde polymer compounds (similar to formaldehyde) that are created when frying with vegetable oils. Trans fats were created for their stability and to control this problem. The focus on trans fats has shadowed the fact that frying foods in vegetable oils is even more toxic than frying them in trans fats, which is what is happening now across the world, from French fries to stir-fries. The only fry-worthy fats are the very saturated types (lard, goose fat, palm oil, coconut oil and butter) but these are so out of favour with the food industry and so expensive that they are rarely used. Ultimately the hotter the fat (even when saturated), the more likely it is to create toxic pro-inflammatory compounds such as AGEs (advanced glycation end-products) and nitrosamine. My recommendation is to use saturated fats to shallow fry and be mindful to keep the heat down (smoking is not a good sign!) while avoiding excessive browning.

3. Excess omega-6 to omega-3 ratio in diet

Research on omega-3 essential fatty acids has dominated the media for the past 10 years. Omega-3 fatty acids are found in the fat of oily fish, in the meat, eggs and milk of grass-fed animals and in some oily seeds and nuts such as flax, hemp and walnuts. Their crucial role in brain/mental health, learning and inflammation control has propelled omega-3 to celebrity status and the phrase is now used as a potent advertising incentive – from 'omega-3 enriched' eggs to salad dressing. The subject is a bit more complicated than that and requires deeper examination and understanding. Omega-3 essential fatty acids (EFAs) are a class of fatty acid and they are not all the same.

Non-animal-sourced omega-3 (ALA) has to be converted into an active form before it can be used by the body. This can be problematic if the enzyme responsible is deficient – as frequently appears to be the case – and is a strong argument in favour of taking animal-sourced omega-3 (EPA and DHA), in the form of a supplement or in the diet. However, the omega-3 content in animal products varies dramatically, depending on how the animal was fed. A farmed salmon will have very little, if any at all, while grass-fed cattle will have a lot. An omega-3 supplement will be good quality only if the oil is very fresh (omega-3s are notoriously unstable and sensitive to light) and sourced from a clean fish that has not been exposed to pollutants such as mercury.

One of the relevant factors in inflammation is the ratio between omega-6s (commonly found in oleaginous seeds and seed oils) and omega-3s. Since the introduction of 'vegetable oils', made from soya, corn, canola/rape and cottonseeds by the food industry in the early 1920s, our diet has become heavily biased towards omega-6 fatty acids and is thought to be the reason why our omega-3 to -6 ratio is now so out of balance, contributing to chronic inflammation. This is another convincing argument for avoiding vegetable oils and processed foods altogether, rather than getting overly concerned about omega-3 to -6 ratio. Ideally, source your omega-3-rich animal products by carefully selecting organic or wild meat, dairy, eggs and fish. If I have to recommend an omega-3 supplement, I prefer those from sustainably sourced fish or krill that are regularly tested for contaminants, and packaged in a way that limits oxidation, as omega-3 fatty acids are notoriously unstable.

4. Sugar

By raising blood sugar, dietary sugars contribute to tissue damage and hardening (glycation) and cause inflammation. Normally, insulin is quickly released to control blood sugar peaks, limit tissue damage and force the sugar out of the blood. Unless the sugar is required for intense energy (eg exercise), insulin will stimulate fat synthesis (in particular intra-abdominal fat) to deal rapidly with the excess blood sugar. When fat cells become overly stretched by fat storage in response to regular and excessive blood sugar, they will burst and/or start to develop insulin resistance – a precursor to hyperglycaemia (excessive blood sugar) and diabetes, thus contributing further to raised blood sugar and tissue damage. Burst fat cells cause an immune response and chronic inflammation.

WOMEN

in the western world apply up to

515

DIFFERENT CHEMICALS

to their body every day.

Only **11%** of them
have been tested for safety and the
majority of those have been found to be

TOXIC, CARCINOGENIC AND/OR

HORMONE DISRUPTERS.

5. Free radicals

These characteristically contribute to the parched skin of over enthusiastic sunbathers and the dull, wrinkled complexion of heavy smokers. However cigarettes and extreme sunshine are not the only culprits to watch out for when it comes to damaging free radicals. The worst dietary and lifestyle habits that generate oxidative stress are:

- **Roasted, toasted, blackened or barbecued foods:** the browner the colour, the more AGEs (advanced glycation end-products) are present in the food. Aptly named, they are formed when, under intense heat, protein and sugar bind together. They speed up oxidative damage to cells and can alter genetic expression. This chemical process is also thought to be involved at cellular level in the hardening of tissues and arteries. AGEs are best kept to a minimum in the diet.

- **Sugars, especially added processed sugars and lactose (from milk):** sugars tend to contribute within the body to the formation of endogenous AGEs. Endogenous AGEs are thought to be largely responsible for the tissue damage that occurs with high blood sugar and to cause the common complications of diabetes (cardiovascular and kidney disease, nerve damage and blindness).

- **Nitrosamines:** nitrosamines are found in some cosmetics, pesticides, and in most rubber products. Known carcinogens, they are also present in drinks and processed foods, especially beer, processed meats (ham, turkey slices, etc), pickled fish and some factory-made cheeses. Deep-frying will also contribute to the formation of nitrosamines. Currently this is a hot topic for the meat-processing industry as governments are trying to limit nitrites (precursors to nitrosamines) that are used as preservatives. Tobacco is particularly high in nitrosamines and e-cigarettes also contain significant levels, bringing into question their safety. Nitrosamines are not generally added to cosmetics but may form after manufacturing. Particularly relevant precursors are cocamidopropyl betaine and cocamide DEA, which are used as emulsifiers in skin milks and lotions.

THE INTERNAL FACTORS THAT CONTRIBUTE TO CHRONIC INFLAMMATION

1. Fat cells: the enemy within

Not all fatty tissues are the same and when it comes to chronic inflammation, intra-abdominal fat is the type that directly causes the most problems. Both excess sugar and stress stimulate intra-abdominal fat deposits. Of all the contributing factors abdominal fat is *the* most significant marker for inflammation, pain and auto-immune diseases. It is not always accompanied by excess weight (high BMI) or obesity. Many people refer to charts that give a generalised ideal weight for our height and age, and feel reassured that they appear to have a 'healthy weight', yet they carry excess abdominal fat. In fact, measuring waist circumference is a far more accurate way of assessing our physiological age, because with excess intra-abdominal fat comes ageing of tissues and loss of organ function. By getting rid of abdominal fat you will literally be turning the clock back on your physiological age.

2. Vitamin D deficiency

Vitamin D is ubiquitous and useful in just about every cellular activity. It is thought to participate in genetic encoding and replicating. Consequently and as a result of a recent meta-analysis, deficiency in vitamin D was identified as the single relevant factor in early morbidity from all diseases. Vitamin D deficiency is also frequently seen in people with chronic (inflammatory) disease and I recommend that you check your vitamin D blood levels if you suffer from inflammation, chronic symptoms or allergies (see text box on vitamin D for more details).

3. Oestrogen toxicity

Oestrogen tends to promote inflammation when present in excess. This is possibly why a lot of auto-immune diseases (lupus, rheumatoid arthritis, etc) are more prevalent in women. Oestrogen toxicity has become a feature of our environment because many pollutant chemicals (plastics in particular) closely resemble oestrogen and will bind to oestrogen receptors. This interferes with oestrogen levels by suppressing the signals to stop producing it. There is a close correlation between increasing levels of environmental oestrogenic pollutants and chronic diseases. Oestrogens are detoxified through the liver and can be synthesised by gut bacteria, so both those factors must be addressed when looking at oestrogen toxicity. Fatty tissues also generate oestrogen and excess weight is a marked contributor to oestrogen toxicity as well as inflammation.

4. Gut permeability

At the interface between external and internal processes the skin and gut lining are crucial surfaces where delicate exchanges take place between the environment and our tissues. Their integrity is essential in controlling systemic inflammation. Local irritation of the gut from inappropriate foods or bowel flora leads to micro-damage of the intestinal barrier and thinning of the delicate mucous layer. This will contribute to the seeping through of alimentary protein and bacterial toxins into the bloodstream.

To maintain intestinal integrity:

◆ **Avoid emulsifiers found in processed foods:** these have been shown to literally dissolve the protective layer of mucus and open the way for bacteria to damage the gut lining.

◆ **Avoid excess gluten:** gluten is a protein found in wheat (and wheat derivatives like spelt and Kamut), barley and rye. Modern wheat is particularly high in gluten because it makes bread 'doughy' – a quality especially appreciated by some commercial bakers. Research shows that the blood-brain barrier – the barrier that keeps poisons out of the delicate brain tissues – is negatively affected by gluten. Gluten also makes the intestinal lining more permeable, which allows proteins to get into the bloodstream, where they don't belong. This sensitises the immune system and promotes inflammation and auto-immunity, both of which play a role in the development of chronic inflammation.

◆ **Avoid excess casein:** similar in structure to gluten, casein is the sticky protein found in milk and dairy products. It is especially concentrated in hard cheeses. Casein and dairy products as a whole are best eaten in moderation. They often contribute to intestinal micro-damage whether from excess lactose fermentation or casein intolerance. Casein has also been named as a trigger for the production of insulin-like growth factor 1 (IGF-1), which is often cited as a possible cancer-stimulating factor.

◆ **Avoid alcohol:** alcohol is a known intestinal irritant that erodes the fragile mucous layer and gut lining.

◆ **Avoid food allergies:** food allergies and sensitivities are specific to the individual. Be particularly mindful of proteins such as gluten (in barley, wheat and rye) and casein (in dairy). Soya, eggs, nuts and pulses can also cause allergies and contribute to chronic low-grade micro-damage of the bowel wall and fuel chronic inflammation. The latter is also in large part controlled by our friendly bacteria and how they react with the food we eat.

◆ **Cultivate your friendly bacteria:** gut flora are fundamental to immune and digestive health. Healthy bowel flora will prevent pathogens invading the protective mucous layer and gut membrane. They directly contribute to healthy digestion.

COLOUR THERAPY: A QUICK GUIDE TO ANTIOXIDANTS

Antioxidants donate electrons without themselves becoming unstable and in so doing protect our cells from the unavoidable damage of oxidation. They work together as shields and the more we have on our side, the better.

VITAMIN D

Vitamin D is synthesised by the skin when exposed to sunlight (UVB), but not if the day is overcast – or in winter when the angle at which the sun hits the earth is too shallow. In order to produce adequate amounts of vitamin D at least 50% of the skin has to be exposed to the sun for roughly 25 minutes. For the average UK resident this almost never happens. There are small amounts of vitamin D in fish oil, liver and egg yolks – and milk fat if the cow has fed on grass and spent time outdoors.

Most of us are deficient in vitamin D. Statistical analysis shows that we could cut our risk of death by 50% by ensuring adequate levels. Only a blood test will determine if you are deficient.

Optimum levels are between 50 ng/ml (125 nmol/L) and 70 ng/ml (175 nmol/L). In the case of chronic disease it may be better to aim for 100 ng/ml (250 nmol/L). More than 100 ng/ml is excessive. If you are unable to go in the sun regularly keep your levels topped up by taking between 3000 IU (75 mcg) and 5000 IU (125mcg) of vitamin D3 per day relative to your weight and size. It is essential to take vitamin K2 (200mcg/day) with it to prevent disruption to your calcium metabolism. Look for a combined supplement.

Carotenoids

Carotenoids are found widely in plants, algae, yeast and bacteria that depend on photosynthesis; they are present in pigments from red to purple and there are more than 600 types. The more intense the colour, the richer the carotenoid content. Carotenoids protect us against sun-radiation damage. Some can be converted to vitamin A in the liver and so are referred to as pro-vitamin A. The conversion depends on an enzyme in the body, which can be deficient or impaired. In this case people tend to gain a slightly orange hue (especially on hands and feet) after eating a lot of orange-coloured fruit and vegetables, and they need to be mindful not to become vitamin A deficient. Generally, carotenoids contribute to a healthy 'rosy' complexion. In the animal kingdom they are responsible for the pink colour of flamingoes, which feed on krill rich in a type of carotenoid (astaxantin from the bacteria and plankton they in turn consume), and for the intensity of egg yolk (zeaxanthin from corn in particular). The following are some of the best-known and researched carotenoids found in food; they work in synergy to give the characteristic colour of individual foods and their antioxidant capacity also varies. This is why research[1] on isolated synthetic beta-carotene supplements is so disappointing. Carotenoids should

1 http://www.nejm.org/doi/full/10.1056/NEJM199404143301501

be viewed as a whole family and appreciated as a potent and complementary source of valuable antioxidants. They are stable in heat and sometimes, because of their limited solubility, even benefit from cooking and the presence of oil. Fruit and vegetables are rich in carotenoids; they can also be found in meat, fish, eggs and dairy products, depending on the animal's diet.

- **Alpha-carotene:** common green-coloured pigment found in all green fruits and vegetables (lamb's lettuce, kale, spinach, peppers, etc). Also found in lesser amounts in orange-coloured fruits and vegetables such as carrots, squash, apricots and mangoes.
- **Beta- and gamma-carotenes:** characteristic yellow/orange pigments found in yellow fruits and vegetables such as carrots and squash, as well as tomatoes, raspberries and red peppers.
- **Zea-carotene:** purple pigment in corn, sweet potatoes and most fruits.
- **Cryptoxanthin:** deep-red pigment in red fruits, vegetables and spices.
- **Lycopene:** also red-coloured, lycopene is found in particularly high concentrations in tomatoes and is well documented for its benefits against prostate cancer. For maximum benefit cook the tomatoes in a little coconut oil and let the juice simmer until it concentrates. As little as one tsp per day of concentrated tomato paste has been shown to be protective against prostate cancer, but make sure that you prepare it yourself or buy it in glass jars. The acidity in tomatoes makes them corrode their packaging and we end up consuming unwanted toxic chemicals (aluminium and BPA in particular).
- **Zeaxantin and astaxantin:** orange-coloured and involved in the characteristic colour of salmon, trout, krill, shrimp, egg yolk. Paprika, spinach and berries are rich sources.
- **Lutein:** intensely yellow, lutein is also found in green-coloured foods such as spinach, parsley, kale etc and in most fruits.

Zeaxantin, lutein and astaxantin are extensively researched because of their specific protective function against oxidation and sun damage to the retina in the eye. They are particularly useful in the treatment and prevention of macular degeneration and similar eye conditions.

- **Canthaxanthin:** brown/red pigment specifically found in mushrooms.
- **Crocetin:** yellow/orange pigment uniquely found in saffron. It has been shown to have potent neuro-protective effects and to improve sleep.

Flavonoids

Along with carotenoids, flavonoids are antioxidants that readily donate electrons and prevent excessive free-radical damage. However flavonoids play a more specific role against (chronic) inflammation. They are being extensively researched in the light of recent discoveries about the negative impact of chronic inflammation on the development and outcome of degenerative diseases such as Alzheimer's, MS, diabetes, certain cancers and cardiovascular diseases.

Flavonoids are intensely coloured and a sub-category of "polyphenols" – the compounds broadly responsible for the medicinal properties of plants and foods. Many medicines contain modified plant polyphenols as active ingredients. They are part of the plant's immune system offering protection against bacteria, fungal infections, viruses and genetic aberrations. Those remarkable properties make polyphenols, and more specifically flavonoids, valuable therapeutic agents against allergies, infections and inflammation. They also support detoxification, hormonal balance and genetic expression.

Because flavonoids are produced by plants in response to (immune) challenges, wild or organic plants are far richer in flavonoids than cultivated and sprayed varieties. This is another reason to choose organic. Flavonoids are difficult to synthesise, although labs are desperately trying to imitate them in order to patent them, but health benefits are consistently greater when flavonoids are obtained directly from plants.

The following are examples of a few well-known types of flavonoids:

◆ **Anthocyanins:** purple/blue-coloured flavonoids. Red grapes and blueberries are a rich source and they can also be extracted from pine bark. An anti-ageing 'must-have', anthocyanins are especially useful in protecting collagen and subcutaneous tissues from sagging, are neuro-protective and useful for the eyes.

◆ **4-oxo-flavonoids:** quercetin is the best known and is a great anti-inflammatory. Supplements can be used against allergies and in the management of diabetes. It is found in red onions, sorrel, capers, watercress, dill and buckwheat.

◆ **Citrus bioflavonoids:** found mostly in citrus fruits (especially the pith) and useful for capillary health and micro circulation. They work in synergy with vitamin C.

◆ **Isoflavonoids:** found in most pulses but especially soya, alfalfa and red clover. They are known for their oestrogenic properties and used to relieve menopausal symptoms. Their oestrogenic properties depend upon proper fermentation in the gut. For this reason only eat fermented soya products from non-GM organic soya. Tempeh, miso and tamari are the better known fermented soya products.

The following are not flavonoids, but are notable polyphenols:

+ **Catechins:** found in green tea, wine and raw cacao, they are a hot topic because research has shown that they offer powerful inflammation and cardiovascular protection. They have a positive action against histamine (in case of allergies) and help with lead detoxification. They contribute to anti-ageing by supporting liver (detox) enzymes potentiation (cytochrome P450, glutathione, and superoxide-dismutase) and seem to work at relatively low doses. Unfortunately black tea is not a good source of catechins, but as few as three cups of organic-quality green tea a day have been shown to have cardiovascular benefits.

+ **Ginkgo flavone glycosides (from ginkgo), curcumin (from turmeric root) and silymarin (from milk thistle):** other examples of well-documented polyphenols with cardiovascular and hepato-protective properties used to support liver detox and anti-ageing. The most effective forms of milk thistle and ginkgo are in alcohol (liquid extracts), while curcumin needs fat for better absorption. The extraction method can multiply bio-availability by a factor of 10 so is important to take into consideration – as is the origin of the plant itself.

+ **Resveratrol:** much discussed as the magic ingredient in red wine and cacao; it is radio-protective, a potent liver detox support that can be used alongside chemotherapy, and has been shown to be anti-cancer, anti-inflammatory and protective of the cardiovascular and nervous systems. For therapeutic use, supplement with resveratrol extracted from grape seeds. Supplement content ranges from 20 to 500mg. It is generally agreed that resveratrol is more potent at lower doses and I recommend that you start with no more than 100mg/day.

+ **Glutathione:** a key antioxidant heavily involved in liver detoxification. It plays a major role in hormonal balance, and in neutralising all those nasty chemicals we have to deal with on a daily basis. The more efficient and plentiful our glutathione pathway is, the better our detoxification. It offers strong protection against cancer and ageing. Glutathione comes partly from food (especially asparagus, walnuts and avocados) but it is fragile and easily destroyed by cooking. The majority is synthesised from three amino acids (L-cysteine, L-glutamic acid, and glycine). To boost glutathione levels you can take the supplement N-acetyl-cysteine (NAC) and whey protein, drink fresh raw, green vegetable juices and practise coffee enemas.

SPICE IT UP!

TURMERIC

is one of the most researched culinary spices. It has over

600

Potential **PREVENTATIVE &**
THERAPEUTIC applications,
as well as

175

Distinct beneficial
PHYSIOLOGICAL effects.

http://www.greenmedinfo.com/blog/science-confirms-turmeric-effective-14-drugs

THIRD TARGET: GUT FLORA

"The best time to make friends is before you need them."
ETHEL BARRYMORE

MAKING FRIENDS OF OUR TINY WARRIORS

Bowel flora, or gut bacteria, are fundamental to health. Gut bacteria can transform metabolites into poisons or neutralise a toxin such as lead. Types and levels of gut bacteria have been shown to be determinant in the outcome of many diseases, such as colon cancer, diabetes and liver disease. They have even been shown to influence the likelihood of developing cirrhosis in case of alcoholism[1]. They can regulate many specific gene expressions; in infants, for instance, the lactic acid bacteria present in milk stimulate lactase, the enzyme responsible for digesting lactose (milk sugar). Gut bacteria are implicated in food behaviour, cravings and susceptibility to weight gain. They are connected to mood and mental health and they are seemingly sensitive to our own stress levels. We simply cannot ignore the fact that our evolution and survival are intrinsically connected and dependent on their existence.

WITH A LITTLE HELP FROM OUR FRIENDS

Our intestinal flora originated from our mothers; on our way down the birth canal we encountered and collected our first hefty dose of bacteria. Then we collected a few more different species from our mother's skin and milk, and they began to interact with our specific bacterial environment. During the first 18 to

1 http://www.ncbi.nlm.nih.gov/pmc/articles/PMC3211517/

24 months of life delicate relationships formed between the different resident gut bacteria, the gut immune tissues (GALT) and the various organisms (Gram negative/pathogenic bacteria, viruses, fungi and spores) we encountered as part of our hand to mouth exploration of our surroundings. A child's immune system is largely affected by the mother's flora and matures as it becomes exposed to dirt and pathogens. Children raised in overly sterile environments tend to develop more allergies and infections later in life than those brought up on farms with a more robust attitude to dirt and cleanliness.

Very quickly strains of our 'commencing' bacteria organise themselves into colonies and become established. Although our flora can evolve and be seriously influenced by diseases, medications and diet, those original strains remain dominant throughout our life. The implication being that a less than optimal gut flora in the mother will tend to be passed on to her children.

Although there are bacteria all over our body, the bowel flora is our 'bacterial stock'. The appendix, conveniently tucked out of the way, is our back-up reserve in case of severe flora disruption from diarrhoea and gastro-enteritis. Some strains do better in the mouth, while others thrive in the vagina or on the skin. Even within the gut there are huge variations in our bacterial landscape, depending on our upper or lower digestive tract, pH and proximity to gut lining and mucous. Intestinal function is related to bowel flora and digestion is a good way to assess the general health of our gut flora. Excessive gas, abdominal sensitivity, heartburn, mucus in the stools, constipation or diarrhoea all benefit from improved bowel ecology. Because of this intimate relationship with our flora, the gut is really part of our immune system and must be considered whenever the immune system is deficient. This is the case in many conditions, from allergies and auto-immune diseases to Alzheimer's, HIV and ME.

Although there are known strains of resident bacteria that are common across human populations, our precise bowel ecology is fairly unique, with more general variations according to diet, climate and ethnic origin.

Bacteria are classified according to their type. The most common are Gram-negative and Gram-positive bacteria. Generally speaking pathogenic types are 95% Gram negative and most probiotic types are Gram-positive. This distinction is reflected in their membrane structure and renders the Gram positive bacteria more susceptible to antibiotics and detergents. Gram-negative bacteria release toxins referred to as LPS (lipopolysaccharides). When produced in large quantities by suboptimal gut flora, LPS cause inflammation and are implicated in chronic inflammatory conditions of the liver, gut, nervous and immune systems. They are associated with the characteristic 'brain fog' caused by dysbiosis (a term applied to diseases and illnesses of the digestive tract).

Types of bacteria can be further classified into species (lactobacillus, staphylococcus, bifido-bacteria, etc); type (acidophilus, aureus, breve, etc); and strains (NCFM, antibiotic-resistant strains, B17, etc). Bacterial classification and identification is extremely complicated. It is a controversial subject that is constantly evolving as the identification of genomes and evolutionary pathways is becoming more precise.

Recent research has even highlighted how the different strains of the same bacteria can produce opposite results, hence the importance of correct bacterial identification. A study on acne showed that only two specific strains of the propionibacterium were responsible for acne, the other 66 strains identified on healthy skin appeared to protect against it. A promising strain was even identified for reducing acne when topically applied[2].

THAT GUT FEELING

Looking after a healthy gut flora is relatively simple and will pay dividends; bringing it back to health can be more difficult. The balance between the different species is regulated by complex mechanisms. A specific strain of bacterium will thrive in a propitious environment only if individual members sense that there are enough of them nearby to either form a colony or, if not possible, to unite and form a dormant 'pod' until circumstances become more favourable. This safety in numbers is poetically referred to as 'quorum sensing' and is one of the ways in which bacteria will opt to reproduce. Reaching that critical mass is crucial but can be difficult once other less desirable organisms are already well established. This can work in our favour when friendly (or probiotic) bacteria are strongly implanted and prevent pathogens thriving, or it can mark the beginning of a downward spiral when unfriendly microbes reach the critical number to launch an attack and provoke an infection.

Pathogens will combine with the immune system to create low-grade chronic inflammation of the gut – making the body susceptible to all kinds of contamination. In this way, bacteria will translocate from a damaged leaky gut to the liver and beyond. Lymphatic circulation will become clogged with bacteria, toxins will poison the brain and whole (food) proteins will be free to circulate. Symptoms will range from brain fog and depression to liver congestion, low immunity, fatigue and pain. If left unchecked this situation will irrevocably turn into chronic disease. Leaky gut is the root of many allergies and auto-immune disorders, especially when combined with toxic overload. The effect on the developing nervous system of a young child can be the root of neurological disorders such as autism, ADHD and learning disabilities. The work of Dr Natasha Campbell-McBride[3] has been instrumental in demonstrating the validity

2 http://www.ncbi.nlm.nih.gov/pubmed/23947673
3 http://www.doctor-natasha.com/

of the connection between child behaviour, food allergies, toxicity and gut flora. An increasing number of babies born today also have compromised gut flora, setting the stage for a number of potentially serious health problems, including a heightened risk of allergies and vaccine damage. This is made worse by foetuses now being irrevocably exposed to toxic molecules and environmental poisons. An investigation by the Environmental Working Group (EWG) in 2005 revealed the presence of 287 different toxins in the umbilical cord blood of babies[4]. Cleaning out the toxic burden and improving gut health before getting pregnant is not only beneficial for fertility and for the woman's health; it will optimise the chances of her baby thriving mentally, psychologically and physiologically for the rest of his or her life.

LOVE YOUR FRIENDS

Prevention is always better than cure. Our immune system is incapable of defending us without the help of a healthy probiotic population. To encourage strong and supportive bacterial colonies avoid the following as much as possible.

Antibiotics: although potentially life-saving, antibiotics should be reserved for emergency use, yet they are still overly prescribed by medical and veterinary practitioners. Antibiotics have been in existence only since 1928 and already they are losing their potency, with pathogens fast developing resistance. This should be ringing some very loud alarm bells instead of a murmur. There are other ways to control pathogens when they are not life-threatening. Many herbs and plants are strongly antibiotic, notably garlic, thyme, oregano and cinnamon. Since 1915 medicine has also known about bacteriophage viruses that can target and kill pathogenic bacteria, yet they have generally been ignored. Antibiotic prescriptions are especially damaging to the gut flora of children.

Medications: although less significant than antibiotics there are other medications that interfere with our probiotic bacteria population, notably oral contraceptives, non-steroid anti-inflammatories (aspirin, paracetamol and ibuprofen) and oral corticoids (cortisone). If you have to take this type of medication ensure that you look after your gut flora by regularly taking a probiotic supplement.

Triclosan, bleach and quaternary ammonium compounds (QACs): these are the active ingredients in those "99.99% destruction" sprays, detergents and antiseptic hand washes. They are of grave environmental concern and are contributing to the "new superbug" strains of bacteria. (Have you ever wondered about the 0.01% that's left with a perfectly clean slate to thrive?). The notion that

---

4 http://www.ncbi.nlm.nih.gov/pmc/articles/PMC2867352/

ORAL HYGIENE: HOW TO BE SELECTIVE ABOUT THE BACTERIA IN YOUR MOUTH

The biofilm we call dental plaque is produced by (Gram-negative) bacteria under certain conditions and in response to various threats such as extreme variations in mouth pH, the regular use of antiseptic mouthwash or antibiotics. In this way biofilm can prevent the killing agent(s) penetrating through to the live bacteria, keeping them safe and somewhat dormant.

Biofilm sticks and binds to the teeth. It builds up easily unless removed with regular (water)-flossing and brushing. Ultrasound (from ultrasonic tooth brushes) effectively breaks down plaque. To avoid making your toothbrush and water flosser breeding grounds for bacteria, soak brushes in hydrogen peroxide, and drain and dry your water flosser after each use.

Plaque itself is not a cause of dental caries unless its pH turns sufficiently acidic to corrode the tooth enamel. This is the result of a shift in the dominant species that make up the plaque rather than a direct consequence of eating acidic foods. The delicate balance between microbes in the mouth can be affected by the food we eat, the chemicals we use to clean our teeth and those

bacteria should be destroyed indiscriminately is preposterous, because of the fundamental balance that exists between the different colonies. Normal soap and water is more than sufficient to control hand to mouth infections like colds or flu. Work surfaces can be cleansed by spraying a 50% distilled vinegar solution scented with lemon essential oil. Hydrogen peroxide can be used on specific areas that need to be sterilised.

Fluoride: occasionally added to tap water, it is found in toothpaste and mouthwash and has dubious benefits for tooth decay and plaque formation; it is not the mineraliser once thought but a common (and toxic) antiseptic. The long-term consequence of a strategy that consists of knocking out both probiotics and pathogens only reinforces the virulence of pathogenic organisms – and fluoride is no exception.

Chlorinated water: chlorine is relatively easy to filter and remove from tap water, but beware of chlorinated swimming pools. Ozone and ultraviolet light (UV) treatments are suitable sterilisers with no environmental impact.

Pesticides and petrochemical residues: found on non-organic fruits and vegetables and are damaging to the desirable and naturally occurring lactic acid we find in our food and drink. Sugar, harsh chemicals (fluoride in toothpaste, chlorhexidine in mouthwash, phosphoric acid in soda) tend to be damaging to the healthy balance of oral bacteria. They affect the more fragile and beneficial types and open the way for their sturdier counterparts to thrive. Better long-term strategies include:

- Alkalising the acidic plaque with bicarbonate of soda. This can be diluted to make a mouthwash or added to your toothpaste.
- 'Oil pulling' with coconut oil – swish for 5-10 minutes every morning with a tablespoon of coconut oil to loosen the plaque and protect the gums and teeth. Make sure to spit out the oil afterwards.
- Chewing on a probiotic capsule containing *Lactobacillus reuteri and Streptococcus salivarius* before sleep. Both organisms readily dwell in the mouth and nasal cavity and have been shown to be effective against plaque, tooth decay and gum diseases, as well as protect against viruses.
- The best toothpastes are free from foaming agents, fluoride and other aggressive chemicals. Choose non-foaming, naturally flavoured toothpaste with as few ingredients as possible. Propolis is an excellent and selective mouth sanitiser that can be used if you already suffer from gum disease.

bacteria that thrive on fresh foods. Irradiation and other preserving techniques used to conserve fruits and vegetables have a similar effect and are usually restricted to non-organic fruits and vegetables.

Glyphosate: the active ingredient in the weedkiller Roundup, which works by specifically blocking important pathways for plants and micro-organisms (the shikimates). These are absent in the animal kingdom and that is the argument used in favour of this supposedly 'safe' agro-chemical. However, bacteria are fully dependent on those synthesising pathways and the environmental impact is potentially catastrophic. Glyphosate has already been shown to contribute to the transmission of bovine botulism and to kill amphibians. Glyphosate residues found on non-organic fruits, vegetables and grains have also been shown to negatively impact on bowel flora and to interfere with liver enzymes (cytochrome P450 in particular) even at relatively low levels.

Evidence shows that glyphosate residue on wheat is partially responsible for the huge increase in coeliac disease (severe gluten intolerance) of the past 10 years[5].

Genetically modified foods: a large proportion of the GM foods produced today are grown from seeds that have been engineered to be resistant to the herbicide glyphosate (Roundup). Those GM seeds produce forage and foods

5 http://www.degruyter.com/view/j/intox.2013.6.issue-4/intox-2013-0026/intox-2013-0026.xml

DIGESTIVE ENZYMES: THE LINCHPIN TO GOOD DIGESTION

Digestive enzymes refer to the chemicals produced by our stomach, liver, pancreas and small intestine. They break down foods into simple absorbable elements and are complemented further by bacterial enzymes. Enzymes control gut pH, absorption rate and the residue left for bacteria, thus actively participating in strain selection. This is because the friendly bacteria tend to be more selective about their food source and thrive in an acid environment.

The more abundant our digestive enzymes, the better the digestion and the healthier the flora. Supplementing your diet with digestive enzymes can be an effective way to support digestion and encourage gut flora. Maintaining and encouraging a healthy pH and preventing protein, starch and fat residues discourages the accumulation of less desirable organisms.

Choose a broad spectrum digestive enzyme supplement that breaks down:
- Sugar, starch and fibre: enzymes include amylase, invertase, sucrase, lactase and cellulase
- Fats: enzymes include bile and lipase
- Protein: enzymes include pancreatin, protase, pepsin and chymotrypsin

Additionally, an enzyme supplement can also contain betaine hydrochloride, a strong acid that stimulates bile production, assists protein breakdown, prevents heartburn and regulates digestive pH.

that still contain a significant amount of the herbicide. Glyphosate negatively impacts gut flora and can still be found in the meat of animals that have been fed forage grown from 'Roundup ready' GM seeds.

Cooking at temperatures above 50°C: organic vegetables generally come with their own healthful package of soil-based probiotics that are easily destroyed by heat – a good argument for eating plenty of raw vegetables.

DON'T ENCOURAGE YOUR ENEMIES

Being sensitive to our friendly flora will ensure that they thrive only if we also avoid encouraging the opportunistic microbes that lurk in and around us, waiting for their big moment. Perhaps the most famous is *Candida albicans* (the yeast responsible for thrush), but there are many more, from methane-producing gut bacteria (known to cause constipation) to yeasts, fungi and parasites (the more

BARELY
HUMAN?

∎∎∎∎∎∎∎∎∎∎∎∎∎∎∎∎∎∎∎∎∎∎∎∎∎∎∎∎∎∎∎∎

Just before we are born the genetic material we carry is 100% human. By the time we have made it through the birth canal we've picked up a considerable amount of

NON-HUMAN DNA
from bacteria.

In just

2 YEARS
we go from carrying

100% HUMAN
TO 10% HUMAN DNA

http://www.greenmedinfo.com/blog/science-confirms-turmeric-effective-14-drugs

'FODMAP' FOODS TO CONTROL GUT FERMENTATION

Research on the interaction between sugars present in food and bacterial fermentation has led to a theory that avoiding certain types of sugar can control bloating, flatulence and fermentation. This can be a useful strategy as part of a gut-rebalancing programme. Avoiding all FODMAP foods (see below) is probably unnecessary and in my experience strict avoidance becomes less relevant as gut health and bowel flora improve. Because gut flora also adapts to diet, reintroduce FODMAP foods slowly and gradually once you see a marked improvement in your bowel symptoms rather than continuing to strictly avoid them. These foods are full of antioxidants and supportive of a healthy gut flora, and often being mindful of quantity is all that's required to keep gut microbes in check. The acronym FODMAP refers to the various fermentable sugar-like molecules found in food:

- **Fermentable** by gut bacteria. Even friendly bacteria can cause fermentation. However the overall result on gut health is a matter of balance between colonies, their interactions with the food we eat and the state of the gut. Finding which and how much of those fermentable molecules cause us trouble is a matter of experimentation. Start by becoming aware of the type and where they are found.

- **Oligosaccharides** include fructans, galactans and fructo-oligosaccharides (FOS). They are found in wheat, barley, rye, onions, leeks, garlic, shallots, artichokes, beetroot, fennel, pulses, pistachios, cashew nuts, pulses and chicory root.

- **Disaccharides** include table sugar and lactose in dairy milk.

- **Monosaccharides** include glucose and fructose. Only when a food contains more fructose than glucose is it particularly susceptible to fermentation because the imbalance in sugars delays absorption. This is the case in apples, pears, watermelon, cherries, mangetout, agave syrup and honey.

- **Polyols** are used in 'diabetic foods' and include sorbitol, mannitol, xylitol and maltitol. They are found naturally in prunes, watermelons, nectarines, peaches, apricots, mushrooms, cherries, cauliflower and coconut.

obvious of our unwelcome guests). These organisms tend to thrive on sugar and specific sugar-like molecules. Their spread is controlled by our digestive enzymes and by the overall balance between the different colonies that interact and support each other. Specific pathogenic strains of microbes or parasites may need to be identified via a stool test to be eliminated.

The following can be useful against unwanted gut pathogens:

Garlic: the allicin in garlic is a strong antibacterial, antifungal and antiparasitic. Garlic has well-documented anti-inflammatory and cardio-protective properties. It can also be used as a supplement or as a tincture in an enema.

Oregano oil: the essential oil of oregano is a powerful antifungal and antibacterial. It is effective against the troublesome *Clostridium difficile* and even has potential for healthy gut micro-flora[6]. It is sold in capsules in order to enrich the lower intestine where the troublesome microbes tend to dwell. Take oregano oil capsules for no longer than five weeks at a time to avoid developing resistance.

Caprylic (octanoic) acid: extracted from coconut oil and abundant in human milk, it has excellent antifungal properties and is effective against many gut pathogens including the infamous *Helicobacter Pylori* responsible for most duodenal and stomach ulcers[7]. Start with a low dose to avoid adverse reaction to the destruction of Gram-negative bacteria and the release of toxins (LPS) as a result. Gradually increase from 1500mg to 2500 mg per day, divided into three doses, and preferably not with food

L-glutamine: an amino acid that fuels the very cells that line our gut (epithelial cells). It can effectively support the health of the digestive tract lining and support gut immunity and integrity.

Proteolytic enzymes: the most common is pancreatin or, for a vegetarian equivalent, papain from papaya. Take two or three times a day between meals.

FRIENDLY FOODS

We may be dependent on our gut flora but they are relying entirely on us for food. Give them what they need to thrive and they will contribute to our health and wellbeing. Apart from preventing toxin-producing pathogens from developing, probiotics also participate in the synthesis of protective vitamins and short-chain fatty acids (SCFAs). Precious SCFAs such as butyrate have been shown to prevent colon cancer, lower cholesterol and increase mineral absorption, and are beneficial in the treatment of inflammatory bowel disease such as Crohn's disease.

Another valuable benefit of probiotic bacteria is their ability to produce phytase – the enzyme that breaks down phytates – which we can't make ourselves. Phytates are common in plant-based foods and are made up of minerals and inositol. Without phytase we cannot access any of these precious nutrients. Inositol is essential for the proper action of several neurotransmitters including serotonin and acetylcholine, which are not only essential in mood and brain chemistry but also help regulate bowel function.

---

6 http://www.ncbi.nlm.nih.gov/pmc/articles/PMC3975404/
7 http://www.ncbi.nlm.nih.gov/pubmed/21830350

PROBIOTIC SUPPLEMENTS: WHAT TO LOOK FOR

To be useful a probiotic supplement needs to guarantee the viability and quantity of its organisms. Usually it will say that at the time of manufacture, it contained a set number of live bacteria. To ensure that a supplement retains its potency it should contain at least 15 billion bacteria, be refrigerated and have a stated sell-by date.

Too many unrelated varieties of bacteria will compete with one another and it is more useful to experiment with only a few strains at a time and evaluate how well they implant in the gut. This will become evident after a few weeks if you notice better stool consistency and frequency, less bloating and flatulence and reduced symptoms of chronic infections such as thrush or cystitis. Having found a compatible probiotic supplement, take it regularly and consistently before food, for six months minimum, to ensure that colonies get established. The following is a guide to the main probiotic strains to look for:

Bifidobacteria (bifidum, longum, lactis, breve and *infantis)* mainly reside in the colon. They help detoxify and protect the bowel and stimulate peristalsis. They produce an array of antibiotics that help keep pathogen populations down.

The types of foods that will support healthy probiotic populations are:

- **Fresh pollen:** contains a multitude of micro-organisms that support healthy and diverse bowel flora
- **Fermented foods:** positively contribute to the diversity of our bowel flora
  Notable fermented products include:
  Natural bio yoghurt and fermented dairy products
  Fermented vegetables, sauerkraut, etc
  Fermented soya products including shoyu, natto, miso and tempeh
  Fermented grains used to make sourdough
  Fermented pulses included in many traditional Asian dishes. This process substantially improves their digestibility and nutritional value
  Fermented butter
  Unpasteurised (apple cider) vinegar
- **Fibre:** consisting of complex chains of carbohydrate (sugars) that are generally non-digestible. However these sugars are fermentable by bacteria and therefore a valuable source of energy for our probiotic population
  There are many different types of fibre, each with individual benefits:
  Cellulose is an insoluble fibre and the main type found in bran. It is useful to bulk out the stools.
  Hemicellulose is found alongside cellulose in fruits and vegetables and

- *Lactobacillus acidophilus* is one of the main residents of the human gut and also dwells in the mouth and vagina. It assists in digestion, particularly milk, and maintains an acid pH that inhibits pathogen growth such as candida.
- *Lactobacillus casei* and *rhamnosus* are particularly well-documented for their anti-inflammatory properties. They are also useful against *Helicobacter pylori* (responsible for the majority of duodenal and stomach ulcers) and against rotavirus infections (colds and flu). They support the lungs and bladder and can also help protect the skin.
- *Lactobacillus reuteri* is a more hardy variety that establishes well in the gut with similar properties to *L. acidophilus.*
- *Lactobacillus gasseri* has been shown to help reduce abdominal fat by an average of 4.6% and to reduce gut permeability to dietary fat[*].
- *Bacillus coagulans* and *Saccharomyces boulardii* have been shown to play a valuable and supporting role to the other probiotic bacteria. They are hardy and resistant to antibiotics. For this reason it is recommended to supplement for shorter times (no longer than three months) and in lower numbers (500 million organisms/day).

particularly in oats. Unlike cellulose, hemicellulose is water soluble and more readily binds to toxins and bile acids. It can slow down carbohydrate absorption and help with blood sugar control.

Pectin is another water-soluble fibre found in fruits, especially citrus. It is very beneficial as it binds to and eliminates heavy metals and neutralises hormone-like toxins (xeno-oestrogens in plastic, water supplies, detergent, etc) and radioactive material. Available as a supplement.

Mucilage is a water-holding gelatinous substance found in psyllium, chia, fenugreek and flax seeds. It has soothing properties and is the active ingredient in aloe vera, slippery elm and marshmallow root.

Alginates are thickening agents found in seaweeds and algae; they bind to radioactive radium and heavy metals.

Lignans are a type of polyphenol (see antioxidant) found alongside fibres in seeds, particularly flax and sesame, and in legumes. They have powerful antibacterial, antiviral and antifungal activity and have been shown to prevent oestrogen- and testosterone-dependent cancers. They can facilitate oestrogen elimination and help bind to oestrogen receptors, thus reducing oestrogen production.

Oligosaccharides (OS): Not exactly fibre, but types of sugars that cannot be digested by the human gut. Notable oligosaccharides are abundant in human milk (galacto-oligosaccharides) where they play a fundamental role in priming a baby's

[*]http://www.nature.com/ejcn/journal/v64/n6/full/ejcn201019a.html

gut and his immunity. Fructo-oligosaccharides (FOS) are found in certain vegetable like artichokes, onions and asparagus. Oligosaccharides are the selective energy source for the *Bifido-bacteria*. Those are unique in their ability to ferment OS and produce the precious short-chain fatty acids (SCFAs) alongside lactate. The cells lining the gut (epithelial cells) are dependent on SCFAs and lactate for their energy, growth and differentiation. Butyric acid is one of the notable SCFAs that has been shown to control bowel inflammation[8].

THE SAD TRUTH ABOUT GM FOODS AND GLYPHOSATE

- The leading GM (genetically modified) crop producers are the United States, Argentina, Brazil, Canada, India and China.
- Spain is the largest producer of GM crops in Europe (20% of Spain's maize production planted in 2013 was GM), followed by the Czech Republic, Slovakia, Portugal, Romania and Poland.
- As of September 2014, 49 GMOs (genetically modified organisms have been authorised by the European Union, including eight GM cottons, 28 GM maizes, three GM oilseed rapes, seven GM soybeans, one GM sugar beet, one GM bacterial biomass, and one GM yeast biomass.
- In 2015 Bulgaria and Scotland voted for a total ban on GM crops.

Aside from the ethical implications and long-term consequences that may arise from the manipulation of life's 'hard drive', there are some very immediate and serious concerns about GM crops. The typical argument that they are an answer to world hunger and an expanding global population under the threat of climate change is a feeble one when you consider that those who may need them most cannot afford to buy the seeds and those who can afford them will pollute our environment and drain world resources further as a consequence.

There are serious questions about the long-term safety of GM food consumption. Already some researchers are making connections with increased risks of cancer but the technology and science is far too recent to be evaluated reliably one way or the other.

Without entering into a polemic, the most immediate concern associated with GM food is increased use of the herbicide glyphosate (brand name Roundup). A large proportion of the GM seeds sold today have been modified to be resistant to it so that entire fields can be sprayed but only the weeds will die.

Monsanto is the leader in this technology with its patented 'Roundup Ready'

8 http://www.ncbi.nlm.nih.gov/pubmed/1612357

corn, cotton, canola, soybean and sugar beets. By using these seeds, farmers around the world are looking to increase yield by reducing weed growth but are creating glyphosate-resistant superweeds instead. According to the Institute of Science in Society the US is the worst affected, with 13 different glyphosate-resistant weed species in as many as 73 different locations.

Glyphosate use in the US has doubled between 2001 and 2007. Although it is used as a weedkiller it is also sold as a desiccant for ordinary crops. Farmers are encouraged to plan, harvest and kill their crops with one application to improve uniformity. Together with Roundup Ready GM seeds (about 20% of the glyphosate migrates out of the plant's roots and into the surrounding soil), this practice is largely responsible for the contamination of soil and water by this far-from-safe chemical.

Although glyphosate safety claims are based on its selective targeting of a specific metabolic pathway (the shikimates) that humans don't possess, this doesn't make it safe. It has been found to be a probable carcinogen to humans and a lethal poison to fishes, invertebrates, algae and bacteria.

The effect on bacteria is particularly worrying because bacteria in the soil control plants' nutrient uptake and affect the quality of the food we grow, but also because the gut bacteria of animals fed on glyphosate-containing GM foods are affected. Just as we are seeing glyphosate-resistant superweeds we are now seeing superbugs in cattle. For example, toxic botulism is now becoming a more common cause of death in dairy cows because the beneficial organisms that naturally controlled the disease are being affected by the glyphosate in the feed. The sensitive gut flora of humans are likely to be affected in the same way.

Glyphosate-resistant GM crops are grown for cattle and animal feed or for the processed food industry. If you eat intensively raised (CAFO) meat and/or processed foods (including bread, breakfast cereals etc) you are most likely consuming GM ingredients. Only by eating 100% organic products can you be sure that you are eating GM-free: while manufacturers must indicate GM ingredients on food labels by law, they are not obliged to if the GM ingredients form less than 0.9% of the total or if the food became accidentally contaminated. The GMO compass provides up-to-date resources.[9]

9 http://www.gmo-compass.org/eng/news/

FOURTH TARGET: SUGAR DEPENDENCE

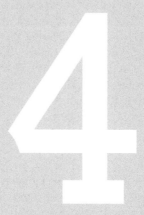

"The mind is not a vessel to be filled but a fire to be kindled."
LAO TZU

BURNING FAT FOR A CHANGE

The energy we require to move, think, digest and generally stay alive can come from carbohydrates sugar), protein or fat. Depending on the fuel we are burning, the effects on tissue ageing are very different. Sugar-burning is a fast process that requires a constant and even supply of sugar to stoke the fire. It is very difficult to control the precise amount of sugar calories to match energy expenditure unless we eat frequently. This is impossible in practice. Blood sugar will go up when we have just eaten, and go down under the influence of insulin soon after. Rapid insulin response is critical to avoid raised blood sugar lasting too long because of the damaging (ageing) effects of sugar on tissues. Insulin triggers the conversion of excess blood sugar (glucose) into glycogen, primarily in the liver then the muscles. Those glycogen reserves are easily converted back into glucose, thus contributing to a steady supply of glucose energy for our cells, and brain, in particular. However, there is only so much glycogen you can store at any one time. In practice an office worker who has a muffin in the morning and a sandwich at lunch time will have barely started to tuck into his liver glycogen before he is eating a huge load of blood sugar-raising foods again! This quickly starts to spell trouble. The sugar can no longer be stored and has to be turned into fat for shuttling to the nearest adipose tissues located around the abdomen and internal organs. The more we abuse this system by eating more carbohydrates than we need (from sugar and starchy foods like grains and potatoes), the less efficient it becomes. Fatty deposits become engorged with fat and rebel against insulin trying to force entry (this is aptly referred to as insulin resistance); more insulin is required to shuffle the sugar out of the blood and it takes much longer for excess blood sugar to return to healthy levels, if at all. As the situation deteriorates further, blood sugar levels never quite return to healthy levels, diabetes ensues with the consequence of our tissues ageing.

Fat is the alternative fuel to sugar. As long as the cells have a good supply of oxygen and we are not pushing ourselves beyond aerobic capacity (which does require sugar), we can evenly power on fat. Fat must be converted by the liver into blood soluble ketones capable of fuelling energy-hungry muscles, brain and heart tissues. Ketones can't totally replace all the sugar required by the brain, but they can replace most of it. In fact, ketones have been shown to stimulate brain regeneration, help control epilepsy and improve memory. According to some experts Alzheimer's disease and other brain disorders could even be induced by the constant burning of glucose by the brain, and neurological damage has been partially reversed by inducing ketosis[1]. Fat-burning can never properly kick-in if we are constantly feeding ourselves with sugar and carbs while keeping our glycogen reserves constantly topped up. Sugar will always take priority over fat. Ideally sugar should be kept for the anaerobic (without oxygen) demands of intense effort and sourced from glycogen (muscle sugar) reserves rather than from the blood where it is susceptible to deregulated insulin and causes tissue damage.

There are many advantages to burning fat rather than sugar. We can only store limited amounts of sugar and supplies quickly run out. Fat on the other hand is practically endless. An average 70kg man has enough fat to burn for 40 straight days before running out. This means when we are powering on fat we no longer get the typical energy dips associated with low blood sugar and which lead to cravings, fuzzy thinking, headaches, irritability, anxiety and depression. The difference between sugar and fat is the same as a tanker transporting tons of fuel and having to stop at the petrol station every few hundred miles. When powering on sugar we are carrying huge amounts of energy but are unable to use it. To dig deep and utilise fat not only provides us with an even energy supply, it also means that fatty deposits are reduced, weight is easy to maintain and muscle mass is protected from having to supplement the sugar with proteins whenever it runs low. Ultimately, you know that you are burning fat when you feel calmer, more relaxed, are thinking clearly and no longer feeling sleepy after eating or in the middle of the afternoon.

---

1 http://www.ncbi.nlm.nih.gov/pmc/articles/PMC2367001/

THE SUGAR MYTH

Sugar and more generally carbohydrates (the food category that refers to all that is sweet and/or starchy, from honey and fruits to bread and potatoes) are often thought of as the stuff of life; the energy that powers all creatures big and small. We are often told that our big brain is incapable of fuelling on anything else and that carb-loading is the best way to increase energy supply for sports people. Low carb diets are frequently deemed to be dangerous and sugar is promoted as an essential nutrient. All this contributes to a great deal of confusion and as a result we may be aware that sugar is generally unhealthy but have relaxed views about 'natural' or complex sugars. Yet at a cellular level they are all the same!

Most of the confusion comes from the observation that, in the presence of sugar, the mitochondria (the energy-providing units in cells thought to have

In order to burn fat the mitochondria (where energy is created in the cells) have to make a metabolic conversion, which can be a difficult process – especially if they rarely have to do so. Fat conversion gets easier the more frequently it is required and it is possible to become more efficient at doing it by regularly creating situations that will make it unavoidable.

Reduce sugar dependence and stimulate fat-burning by:
- Reducing sugars, grains and starchy foods (potatoes, bread, rice, etc)
- Experimenting with food timing to regularly empty glycogen reserves and induce ketosis.
- Exercising at high intensity and stimulating the muscles to use up their glycogen. This forces the liver to use up stored fat to make new glycogen.
- Eating coconut and palm oil for their medium-chain fatty acids (MCFAs) content. MCFAs are used directly as 'fat energy' and, unlike other fatty acids, cannot be stored.

MASTERING MITOCHONDRIA WITH INTERMITTENT FASTING

Fat-burning enables you to break free from the tyranny of sugar physiology. This doesn't mean that you will never again be able to look at a carbohydrate; it simply means that your mitochondria are trained to switch from sugar to fat and that running out of sugar no longer sends you into physiological panic.

Manipulating the timing of food is the best way to exercise metabolism to become more efficient at fat-burning. In fact, research shows that it is possible to lose weight without changing diet, calorie intake and activity levels by simply altering the timing of food intake. We just need to allow longer gaps between eating. This

evolved from bacteria) will burn it first. This is regardless of the presence of energy-dense fat. However, this doesn't mean they 'prefer' it over fat. Imagine making a fire with paper, sticks and logs – of course paper and sticks will burn more readily but they will go up in flames and provide no lasting energy unlike the logs.

Looking at our 6 million-plus years of evolution there is a strong argument that until very recently sugar was only seasonally available (typically summer and autumn) and that it readily converts to fat stores in order to see us through the difficult fasting period (winter and spring). In our current times of plenty, storing fat is rarely relevant and our excessive dependence on sugar means that we are gradually exhausting our insulin reserves while creating considerable metabolic disruption. Ultimately circulating sugar will oxidise and damage cells and tissues.

way of eating mimics our ancestors' lifestyle and is more in harmony with our physiology. Prehistoric man hunted for his sustenance every few days and only when he was very hungry. However, we don't have to go that far back –Victorian labourers worked during the day and ate twice daily at either end of their shift. This particular timing, combined with physical activity and improved farming methods meant that for a very short historical period they had a nutrient-rich organic diet while sugar was not yet widely available. Remarkably, this gave rise to a short golden age in the mid-Victorian era when, contrary to popular belief, the health and productivity of the working class was potentially at its best[2], (all the better to deal with the environmental squalor and poor living conditions).

Although reduced calorie intake has statistically been shown to improve longevity, it frequently gives rise to deficiencies, low energy and a reduced metabolic rate. It is also very difficult to sustain and frequently leads to yo-yo dieting. Unlike intermittent fasting, yo-yo dieting signals a forthcoming food shortage and the need to stock up on fat reserves. Intermittent fasting on the other hand signals no food shortage but forces the body to mobilise fatty tissues as soon as sugar reserves are down. It also stimulates the anti-ageing growth hormone (HGH) that promotes lean tissue growth, especially if exercising in a fasting state. While dieting makes you fat, intermittent fasting makes you strong and lean. HGH tends to diminish with age and has a multitude of benefits on bone and muscle density, the immune system and fat mobilisation. HGH keeps you feeling and looking young and is stimulated by intermittent fasting.

Depending on activity, sugar depletion and fat-burning kicks in after about 12 hours without food. In effect this means that by eating your last meal of the

2 http://www.ncbi.nlm.nih.gov/pmc/articles/PMC2672390/

BROWN FAT TO THE RESCUE

Maintaining body heat uses energy and is largely controlled by 'brown fat', a type of mitochondria-rich fatty tissue that's located under the skin. It rubs shoulders with ordinary white fat and is very rich at the top of the spine just below the neck. White fat is a good insulator but it requires very little energy to maintain and does not generate heat. Brown fat on the other hand burns off fat as energy to maintain body heat when we are cold and not shivering.

It behaves like muscle tissues in the sense that it will grow and become stronger the harder it has to work. Unfortunately it can disappear almost completely if never called upon. Working and living in an overly heated environment is a sure way to kill brown fat. However, it is possible to stimulate brown fat synthesis at the profit of ordinary fat by regularly exposing ourselves to cooler temperatures. You can do this by switching off the heating in the bedroom, taking regular cold showers, swimming in cold water, lowering the thermostat at home and wearing fewer clothes.

day at 6pm you could effectively exercise your fat-burning ability while sleeping through most of your fasting period.

For maximum benefits you can extend your fasting time to a 24-hour period by eating once per day for two days a week while fitting some form of exercise into your fasting time. If you regularly practise this intermittent fasting routine not only will fat storage be reduced but so will the number of fat cells.

This metabolic workout has been scientifically shown to reverse ageing using the following health markers:
- Cardiovascular health, cholesterol and circulation
- Pro-inflammatory intra-abdominal adipose tissues
- Insulin sensitivity and diabetic tendencies
- Growth hormone levels

Additionally it has been shown to improve:
- Immunity
- Appetite hormones (ghrelin and leptin)
- Cellular preservation in favour of healthy cells
- Digestive health

As with any type of training you become better at it the more you practise.

With repetition, intermittent fasting becomes easier and the benefits will soon motivate you to continue.

HOW DIETARY PROTEINS CONTROL FAT-BURNING

Besides intermittent fasting, the ratio between sugar (starch included) and protein is also relevant to ketosis and fat-burning. It's possible to force ketosis by simply limiting sugar intake and forcing the body to meet its basic sugar requirements from proteins. This process of glucogenesis takes place in the liver. We need about 130 grams of glucose per day and, if it does not come from food, glucose can only be synthesised from protein. This process requires energy fuelled by ketones from fat. Depending on the amount of protein we eat, glucose can be synthesised from dietary proteins or lean tissues. Obviously it is better to preserve muscles by eating enough protein to meet regular protein requirements (1.6 grams per kilo of body weight) and extra for glucose demand (0.8 grams per kilo of body weight).

If we follow a low sugar diet (less than 100 grams of total sugar per day) with enough protein to cover basic lean tissue requirements and convert into glucose, we can induce permanent fat-burning while maintaining muscle mass. This happens regardless of the total amount of calories consumed and fat consumption is used to fuel ketosis. This type of ketogenic diet was first developed to help against epilepsy in the 1920s and requires that all the sugar comes from vegetables because the minute you eat fruit, starchy vegetables or grains you will go over the ketogenic threshold.

A low carbohydrate diet is a great way to kick-start ketosis and improve fat-burning metabolism but there is a danger that some people become carb-phobic and start to live on fry-ups! This is a very unhealthy interpretation of ketosis and not one I recommend. However, there are many health advantages to reducing carbs and increasing fats and proteins.

Getting the majority of your calories (up to 70%) from fats (not vegetable oils, fried fats or trans fats) rather than from carbohydrates and sugar also trains your metabolism to fuel on fats. Vegetables should make up the bulk of your diet, with sufficient protein to ensure that you maintain the integrity of your lean tissues; and fats from avocados, eggs, butter/dairy, coconut, nuts and seeds for your energy source.

For a healthy interpretation of sugar metabolism versus fat metabolism we should combine the principles of intermittent fasting with those of a diet that favours carbohydrates from vegetables, fruits and pulses rather than processed foods, grains and sugar. Ultimately you need to find what works best for you.

INACTIVITY LEADS TO PREMATURE AGEING EVEN IF YOU EXERCISE

Mechanisation, the internet and television all lead to inactivity. This is one of the greatest health challenges we are facing today. Our circulation depends on lower-limb contraction; our bones and joints rely on interaction with gravity; our neurology needs movement to process information and to integrate learning; our internal organs depend on the activation of the diaphragm and postural muscles. All this is possible only when we move our body frequently and engage our muscles and joints through their full range of motion. Neither sitting nor standing can do that.

According to an article published in *The Journal of the American Medical Association*, individuals who are physically active appear to be biologically younger than those with sedentary lifestyles*. Oxidative stress and inflammation are mentioned as the likely mechanism by which sedentary lifestyles shorten telomeres. Telomeres are genetic materials which get physically shorter with age. Telomere length is a reliable marker of biological age.

Additional studies have also shown that regular gym attendance alone doesn't benefit telomere length unless those people get up and move around regularly as well.

The following will support beneficial fat-burning:

- **A nutrient-rich diet** supports healthy metabolism. Enhance your diet with superfoods and brightly coloured organic fruit and vegetables.
- **Proteins** prevent hunger, preserve lean tissues, participate in ketosis.
- **Sleep** maintains good general hormonal balance. Sleep regulates appetite hormones (ghrelin and leptin) and growth hormone.
- **Medium-chain fatty acids** are abundant in coconut oil. They cannot be laid as fatty tissues and are used as an energy source by the brain.
- **Fibre** regulates appetite, slows down sugar and carb absorption, feeds friendly bacteria in the gut and supports a healthy metabolism.
- **Omega-3 fats** control chronic inflammation which is a major cause of the metabolic syndrome characterised by excessive sugar/carb dependence. They are found in oily fis, flax, walnuts, grass-fed/organic meat, butter and eggs.
- **Healthy gut flora and fermented foods** reduce fat absorption, improve neurotransmitters in the gut and have been shown to influence food cravings and behaviour. Fermented foods help reduce the impact of gut pathogens involved in inflammation and metabolic syndrome.

*http://archinte.jamanetwork.com/article.aspx?articleid=413815

- **Lower ambient temperature and cold exposure** stimulate brown fat synthesis.
- **Berberine** extracted from herbs, including berberis and golden seal, has antibiotic properties. A recent study showed that it is as efficacious as metformin[3] a common drug for type 2 diabetes. In another study, berberine lowered triglycerides by 35.9%, LDL cholesterol by 21%, and total cholesterol by 18%, compared to minimal declines in cholesterol and an increase in triglycerides in the control group. Furthermore, the group taking berberine had lower blood pressure (average drop of 7/5 mm Hg systolic/diastolic) and modest weight and abdominal fat loss[4].
- **Curcumin** is the active ingredient found in turmeric. It has strong anti-inflammatory properties and has been shown to reverse insulin resistance and other inflammatory symptoms associated with obesity and metabolic disorders. Curcumin may also be beneficial for cancer, Alzheimer's disease, rheumatoid arthritis and other chronic disease. For better absorption combine turmeric with ginger and black pepper. Look for a curcumin supplement that will be more concentrated than turmeric. Choose an oil-based standardised extract, combined with black pepper for maximum benefits and absorption.
- **Conjugated Linoleic Acid (CLA)** is in butter made from the milk of grass-fed mammals. CLA has been shown to support fat-burning especially when combined with exercise.
- **Exercise and movement** are statistically more significant to health, longevity and body composition than nutrition. Metabolism is fully dependent on physical activity to be healthy.

The following directly prevent fat-burning:
- **Starch, alcohol, sugar** all contribute to laying down fat stores
- **Trans fats** cannot be processed by the body. They contribute to inflammation and cause damage to arteries and heart tissues. You'll find them described as 'partially hydrogenated vegetable oil' on labels.
- **Toxic chemicals** disrupt hormonal balance, liver detoxification and increase chronic inflammation and immune disruption.
- **Heavy metals** cause the same problems as above but additionally will be particularly disruptive to thyroid function and metabolic rate.
- **Chronic inflammation** contributes to tissue damage and metabolic syndrome. In particular it can target the liver and pancreas and greatly increase the chances of developing diabetes.
- **Stress** increases inflammation and disrupts hormones. Stress isn't

---

3 http://www.ncbi.nlm.nih.gov/pubmed/18442638
4 http://www.ncbi.nlm.nih.gov/pmc/articles/PMC2410097/

just pressure at work, a difficult relationship or sudden change of circumstances; stress hormones are also generated from watching violence, playing video games and not getting enough sleep.

- **Sleeping less than six hours per night** affects hormonal and neurological balance. Sleep helps to regulate appetite and stress hormones and to maintain good levels of serotonin and neurotransmitters responsible for mood, appetite and wellbeing.

EXERCISE AND MAKE IT WORTH THE EFFORT

Exercise is not the antidote to inactivity or a substitute for moving your body regularly. Movement is the antidote to inactivity. Your body depends on movements such as walking, regularly getting up from your chair and generally mobilising your joints for basic functions like digestion, lymphatic drainage and healthy bones. Specific types of regular exercise can enhance your metabolism, target abdominal fat and slow down ageing better and quicker than anything else mentioned in this book.

Exercise can be aerobic or anaerobic:

Aerobic means the energy required will be coming from an oxygen dependent pathway. Most of the time (even when we are sitting and hardly moving) we are in aerobic mode. Moderate activities like walking are also essentially aerobic.

Anaerobic means that energy is sourced without the presence of oxygen. When we exercise and purposely exert energy our muscles combine both aerobic and anaerobic pathways. The more intense the exercise, the more anaerobic it becomes, and the shorter we can sustain it. Typically, high-ntensity workouts such as heavy weightlifting and sprinting are mostly anaerobic and exclusively use sugar as fuel because fat cannot be 'burnt' without the presence of oxygen. This intense effort encourages muscle fibres to use up their glycogen (sugar store). Muscle glycogen quickly runs out in minutes, even seconds, depending on intensity. This forces the liver to draw on its own glycogen reserves. The good news is that to pushing the liver to use up its glycogen will force it to make new glycogen by drawing on the fat that's nearest – the unwanted pro-inflammatory liver and abdominal fat! This is especially true if you eat a protein-rich low sugar meal post workout. Research[5] has shown positive results on diabetes and metabolic syndrome from high intensity exercise. This doesn't mean that less intense exercise has no benefit but it does point to enhanced (abdominal) fat mobilisation with high-intensity exercise. You can instigate fat-burning from a shorter gym session with a higher-intensity workout.

Increase intensity by adding weight. Slow-moving weight-bearing exercises such as squatting and lunges can be high intensity and mobilise several muscle groups.

---

5 http://www.ncbi.nlm.nih.gov/pubmed/22587821

In fact, barbell squatting has been shown to be one of the best exercises to stimulate human growth hormone (HGH), improve bone density and positively affect muscle-to-fat ratio. The slower you move through your squat, the greater the intensity and associated benefits on metabolism and muscle power.

It is also possible to increase intensity by moving more quickly. In this way short bursts of sprinting are better than long endurance marathon running – and less stressful for your joints! Aim to go flat-out for 20–30 seconds and repeat up to eight times during a 20-minute workout. You can sprint by running, cycling or rowing. Rowing is the least likely to cause injury and can be extremely intense.

The intensity of exercise for fat-burning and metabolic benefits is relative to fitness. The fitter you are, the harder you have to work to challenge your metabolism. Heart rate is a rough guide to evaluate where you are on that scale. To be in your peak intensity zone you have to feel that your heart is pumping hard and that you are rapidly getting out of breath. You should not be able to maintain this level of intensity for longer than 45 seconds.

Weight-bearing exercises have the unique advantage of quickly displacing white fat while building muscle mass and increasing brown fat. The greater your muscle mass and brown fat, the higher your basic metabolic rate. This means that you can be burning substantially more calories (200-500 a day more) even when you are asleep! Muscle mass is an age marker; it diminishes as you get older at the profit of (inflammatory) adipose tissues. Building lean tissues is an insurance against ageing.

If the above makes you want to curl up on the sofa, just remember that to be beneficial, exercise doesn't have to be intense, but it must be regular and frequent. Research proves that inactivity leads to inactivity and our physiology adapts to make us lose the basic urge to move. Conversely, reconnecting with our physiological need for movement will make us want to become more active. Just adding movement of any kind is the single most powerful health choice you can make. Start by taking the stairs whenever you can, stretch and stand up regularly when at your desk, walk to the shop, cycle to work and generally become movement conscious.

Numerous studies demonstrate the benefits to be gained from even gentle exercise, on cardiovascular health, cancer and Alzheimer's prognosis as well as arthritis, back pain, diabetes, depression and sleep. You don't have to join expensive gyms, sign up for 10k runs or join classes in dimly lit church halls miles away (unless you enjoy it). You can get a healthy workout by dancing to your favourite music, cleaning the windows, or gardening. Make it fun and purposeful and you won't even notice that you are exercising.

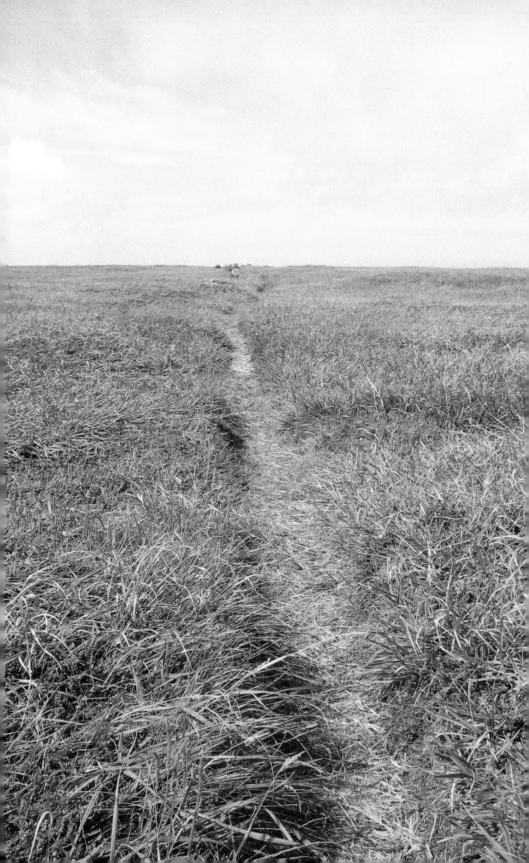

PART FOUR:
MAKE VITALITY LAST

*"Vitality shows in not only the ability to persist
but the ability to start over."*

F. SCOTT FITZGERALD

SHORT-TERM GOALS AND LONG-TERM BENEFITS

No matter how small, if we adopt a particular habit and repeat it regularly, the effects will cumulate over time. Those exponential benefits change us in a way that can either feed into the motivation to continue with living life to the full or confine us to the expectation that with age comes a loss of vitality and wellbeing.

WHEN MAKING ANY TYPESOF CHANGE KEEP THESE FEW PRINCIPLES IN MIND:

- **It is easy to substitute like for like:** start swapping margarine for butter, cooking oil for coconut oil or goose fat, vegetable oils (in shop bought mayonnaise and salad dressings) for home-made vinaigrette using cold pressed olive, flax, avocado, walnut or hemp oil (or a combination), tap water for filtered or spring water and non-organic for organic whenever possible.
- **It is easier to add than take out:** start adding to your regular diet the superfoods, spices, herbs or fresh vegetables that you find appealing
- **Cutting down can be more difficult than cutting out:** if you didn't have those biscuits in the house you probably wouldn't be nibbling them at night when the urge takes you. Be aware that the urge to eat them is rarely at the time of buying them but nonetheless a lot of the foods that we are attached to are, in fact, following an addictive pathway. This means that to begin to control cravings we have to detox and go through a period of abstinence from the main triggers. For some people certain foods/drinks are so addictive that being near them quickly leads to a vicious circle of compulsive behaviour and depression. This is generally the case with sugar but other foods and drinks have hidden ingredients which can have the same effect. Bread, potatoes, crisps, milk and dairy produce, dried fruits, fruit juices, beer and lager, chocolate, wine and of course alcohol as a whole all contain a lot of sugar and can easily become addictive. Sugar substitutes and additives like MSG (monosodium glutamate) found in most processed foods and drinks are also potentially addictive and should be avoided. Recognise your own particular triggers and adopt a strategy that's adapted for you.

If you rarely eat or drink out, this can be a safe boundary and means that you can allow yourself some of those foods if you are in a restaurant, but if eating out is a regular activity you will have to create a 'restaurant strategy'. Choose your restaurants carefully – check menus before you go in – avoid the bread basket and don't order dessert. As a rule of thumb, leave five days apart when consuming a food or a drink that is a potential addictive trigger. Also pay attention to possible side-effects (for instance, eating bread and cheese might trigger some digestive discomfort or alcohol may be a trigger for a poor night's sleep or feeling anxious or sad). This will help you identify not only your behavioural trigger(s) but also your physiological trigger(s) and re-enforce your resolve to avoid them.

- **Get support from friends, family or a professional:** by feeling accountable to another person you are more likely to persevere and they will bear witness to your efforts.
- **If it is unhealthy for you, it is also unhealthy for your family, pets and guests:** don't have it in your house!

THE TEN PRINCIPLES OF CHOICE

Whatever the ingredients for youthful and lasting health, there is no secret; we just have to decide and commit to it. If you are reading this book you probably know this already but you may be wondering where to start. My principles of choice are criteria to help you prioritise and focus on what matters when you are shopping. What we buy and bring home is where it all starts!

Read this list before you go food shopping:

1. **Increase** the amount of vegetables
2. **Avoid sugar** from processed foods and drinks
3. **Limit** alcohol
4. **Eat more fats** and get the facts on 'healthy' fats
5. **Pick quality proteins** to incorporate in your daily diet
6. **Limit** starchy carbohydrates from grains and potatoes
7. **Limit** fruits
8. **Clean up** toxic chemicals from your home and personal care
9. **Incorporate** superfoods in your daily diet
10. **Make** your health your priority and use your buying power wisely

1 INCREASE YOUR INTAKE OF VEGETABLES

Vegetables are low-density high-nutrition foods that are packed with alkalising minerals. They feed our probiotic population and require very little digestion. They help us feel satiated and chewing on raw vegetables contributes to the

WHICH VEGETABLES CONTAIN THE MOST TOXIC CHEMICAL RESIDUES?

According to the Environmental Working Group in the United States:

WITH THE MOST AGRICULTURAL RESIDUES:	WITH THE LEAST AGRICULTURAL RESIDUES:
Peppers	Asparagus
Cherry tomatoes	Avocado
Celery	Leeks
Lettuce (any)	Onions, garlic, shallots
Spinach	Broccoli
Cucumber	Cauliflower
Courgettes	Cabbage, Brussels sprouts
Potatoes	Mushrooms
Green beans and mangetout	Aubergines
	Root vegetables: carrots, beetroot, radishes, parsnips
	Sugar snaps, broad beans

Limit residues: scrub and wash your vegetables in diluted baking soda. Peeling helps but also removes some nutrients.

health of our teeth and gums without raising blood sugar. They come in the most vivid colours and variety of tastes and textures, making them versatile, packed with antioxidants and satisfying to our senses. Aim to make vegetables the central ingredients of a meal so that when you look at your plate more than 60% is made up of vegetables. Eat them cooked and raw, both have their virtues. Vegetables are anti-inflammatory, prevent constipation, keep the skin looking rosy and vibrant and help maintain a healthy weight. Choose organic vegetables whenever possible not just because they will often be richer in nutrients but because they contain fewer toxic chemical residues. As often as possible buy vegetables that are locally produced and in season. Frozen vegetables are the healthiest option when buying vegetables out of season.

If you are not used to eating a lot of vegetables try making juices, purées, flans, soups and smoothies as a way to disguise them and incorporate them more easily into your diet. If you find that eating vegetables gives you gas make sure to take a probiotic supplement and digestive enzymes that include cellulase and phytase with every meal. Introduce vegetables gradually and vary the types. Some ,like the cabbage and onion family, can be worse than carrots and courgettes but digestibility will improve as your probiotic population adapts to your new diet.

2. AVOID SUGAR FROM PROCESSED FOODS AND DRINKS:

If sugar was a medicine and it had to pass the same health assessment for side-effects as a drug it would not be allowed on the market! Sugar leads to rebound hypoglycaemia, fatigue, insulin resistance and eventually diabetes. It is very acidifying and damaging to the tissues. It promotes cardiovascular disease, fatigue (especially after eating), depression and anxiety. It encourages pathogenic bacteria in the gut and raises chronic widespread inflammation leading to pain, allergies, auto-immune diseases and degeneration. Eating sugar feeds into fatty deposits, especially those around the middle. Sugar reduces resistance to stress and infections and directly causes wrinkles, thickening of the skin and tissue ageing. Sugar feeds the reward pathway in the brain in the same way as any hard drug and can be just as addictive yet it is freely and widely available without any health warning.

Wherever it comes from (agave, fruits, coconut, cane, beet, corn) sugar is never a natural product. Sugar and syrups are processed in order to be extracted, fresh fruits and vegetables are not. Honey may be natural but most of the time the bees are fed sugar and the honey is highly processed too. Sugar is used by the food industry to mask other far less palatable chemical tastes, and to sell very cheap and empty foods that no one would want to eat otherwise. The more sugar you consume the less sensitive to its taste you become.

Artificial sweeteners are highly toxic and a useless alternative. They have done nothing to diminish our sugar dependence or reduce obesity, but they come with their own health-damaging (neurological) side effects while continuing to increase sugar cravings and even diabetes. Non-digestible sugars like **stevia** and **xylitol** may be a valuable way to wean yourself off sugar but be aware that they can create bloating.

To improve taste and add interest to food use small amounts of fruit, lucuma (a type of fruit) powder, chopped dates or raisins, vanilla essence or cacao. Ultimately as you develop your sugar awareness and sensitivity you will require less and less of it. It is generally agreed that 25g of sugar per day is a healthy amount which corresponds roughly to five large dates (10 small ones) or one tablespoon of honey.

3. LIMIT ALCOHOL

Alcohol has a specific and metabolic pathway ending up straight as fatty deposits around the liver and heart and an ever-expanding waistline. Because alcohol is also a poison that has to be detoxified by the liver it interferes with detoxification and hormonal balance. In particular it contributes to reduced growth hormone (HGH) and testosterone levels. This directly and negatively impacts on muscle mass and on libido. Regular alcohol consumption is known to interfere with levels of angiotensin, the hormone associated with erectile dysfunction. Long-term drinkers may also experience loss of libido, shrinking of testes, reduction of the size of the penis, reduced sperm formation, loss of pubic and body hair and enlargement of the breasts.

Alcohol also causes erosion of the digestive tract, negatively contributing to chronic inflammation, degenerative diseases and cardiovascular diseases.

To get a clearer picture on the effect of alcohol consumption and cardiovascular diseases, researchers evaluated the cardiovascular health of individuals with a genetic variant of the alcohol dehydrogenase I B gene (a gene marker is typically more accurate than questionnaires used in observational studies). People who have this gene metabolise alcohol faster, which causes symptoms such as nausea and facial flushing. Consequently they are much less likely to drink. Data[1] was gathered from more than a quarter of a million people and showed that individuals with the gene had lower levels of alcohol consumption, better cardiovascular health (lower blood pressure, inflammatory biomarkers, adiposity measures and cholesterol) and reduced risk of developing coronary heart disease. Heart disease risks were directly proportional to how much alcohol people drank. A study investigator wrote: "These findings suggest that reductions of alcohol consumption, even for light to moderate drinkers, may be beneficial for cardiovascular health. Our results therefore challenge the concept of a cardio-protective effect associated with light to moderate alcohol consumption reported in observational studies and suggest that this effect may have been due to residual confounding or selection bias."

Over the years wine has gained the reputation of being a 'healthy alcohol' thanks to its cardio-protective polyphenol content. Grapes such as Chardonnay contain resveratrol and alcoholic fermentation does concentrate it somewhat, but this does not reduce the problems generated by alcohol itself; at best, it neutralises them providing that quantities are small and consumption spread out. The long-term benefits associated with drinking wine are most likely related to other social and lifestyle factors typical of light to moderate drinkers. These are not negligible and make wine consumption something worth doing with appropriate awareness.

---

1. http://www.bmj.com/content/349/bmj.g4164

4. EAT MORE FATS AND GET THE FACTS ON HEALTHY FATS

Fats are essential. They contain precious and essential fatty acids (EFAs). The brain, nervous and hormonal systems have very high EFA requirements. Every single cell in our body needs fats for membrane structure. Fats regulate neurotransmitters and appetite hormones. They help us feel satiated and add palatability to foods. Far from simply being high in calories, they nourish our fat metabolism and help us to be more efficient at mobilising adipose tissue. Eating fats reduces sugar cravings and people who eat nuts regularly have been shown to be less overweight than those who avoid them.

Until the early 1900s most people ate fats from animals in the form of lard, dairy, meat and fish with small amounts of nuts and olives. However, food processing, intensive farming methods and cheap vegetable oils from corn, peanuts, sunflowers, cotton, soya and rape have dramatically altered the dietary balance of saturated/unsaturated fats and between the fatty acids omegas 3, 6 and 9. This situation was compounded even further when poorly led research in the early 70s stated that saturated fats caused heart disease and that (carcinogenic) trans fats and margarine were a suitable alternative.

Despite recognising that trans fats cause disease and that our diet is badly deficient in omega-3 fatty acids, confusion persist, with health authorities and medical practitioners blaming saturated fats and cholesterol for cardiovascular risk. Yet research-based evidence shows that the problem with fat is in the way it combines with sugar and not fat itself.

Our apparent widespread lack of omega-3s, is largely due to (intensive) farming methods. Meat and dairy from animals fed GM corn and/or cereals will have substantially fewer omega-3s than if they had been (even partially) grass-fed.

In practice this means that we need to be selective about the way in which we increase fat consumption. The best animal fats are those that come from organic (grass-fed) or wild fish, meat and dairy. Whole nuts, whole seeds, avocados and olives all provide healthy levels of natural fats and are packed with plenty of additional nutrients like fibre and antioxidants. When fats are extracted from those foods they become more fragile. The more saturated the fat, the less fragile and susceptible to becoming toxic when heated. Goose fat, coconut butter, palm oil and dairy butter are the most stable fats for cooking and baking. The partially saturated olive, avocado and nut oils (like walnut or Brazil nut) are suitable for salad dressings providing they are kept in a dark container and state that they are cold pressed. To ensure that you are getting enough omega-3s and without imbalancing the ratio between 6 and 9, eat oily fish three times a week, you can also choose a quality krill oil supplement and/or eat ground flax or hemp seeds. Aim to avoid the 'vegetable oils' found in supermarkets extracted from soya, corn, rape, peanut, cotton seeds and sunflower and in processed foods. To increase your beneficial fat consumption snack on whole unsalted nuts; make sauces and dressings with tahini (sesame seed butter) or any other nut butter; add coconut butter to your steamed vegetables; substitute the flour in pancakes, breads and muffins with ground almond or coconut flour and enhance your salads with avocados, olives, nuts and seeds.

5. PICK QUALITY PROTEIN TO INCORPORATE IN YOUR DAILY DIET

Protein is a complicated subject almost as confusing as fats, and ethical considerations about provenance, animal welfare and world hunger complicate matters further.

Proteins contain essential building blocks (amino acids) which our body needs to sustain tissue integrity, to repair and to maintain lean body mass. Amino acid requirements will vary considerably depending on physical size, gender, lean body mass percentage and age. Activity, injury and illness increase needs.

Animal proteins (meat, eggwhite, dairy, gelatine) are far better absorbed and their amino acid profile is more harmoniously matched to our own tissues than the vegetable proteins found in nuts, seeds and pulses. There are small amounts of proteins in certain vegetables and in grains but those cannot be regarded as protein foods.

Animal proteins are particularly controversial because of rearing methods and protein's supposed health risks. Rearing methods are not only relevant to animal welfare and to the environment, but also to the quality of the food produced from it. Intense animal farming is not only cruel, it breeds disease, pollutes the environment and produces toxin-laden protein foods with a high carbon footprint. There is nothing healthy about intensive farming. The processed-food industry uses exclusively animals raised intensively – unless it can guarantee provenance and/or organic standards. This means that if you are buying eggs, meat or dairy produce, only those that state they come from free-range, organic or wild animals can be expected not to have been intensively farmed – unless you are buying from a farmers' market and you have spoken to the breeder. Sheep, goats and venison are usually raised on grassland and are an exception. Rabbits can be factory-farmed but are often culled from the wild. Vegetarians are no less cruel than meat-eaters unless they also take the provenance of eggs and dairy into consideration.

Ethic is a powerful argument used by vegans to support their choice to avoid animal products altogether. However this cannot be sustained by health considerations. Animal proteins are in no way a health hazard but they do involve killing animals. Eggs from free-range hens are possibly the furthest removed from

A GROWING
PROBLEM

70% OF ANTIBIOTICS

It's estimated that **70%** OF ANTIBIOTICS are used on livestock as **GROWTH PROMOTERS** in the USA; without them, farmers would have to breed an extra

452m chickens

23m cattle

12m pigs

to supply the voracious demand for meat products. Antibiotics are also used prophylactically to cram even more animals into confined spaces, and have irrevocably found their way into our food chain.

animal killing but for egg production to be sustainable farmers regularly cull old, tired hens to make room for younger more productive ones. Dairy farming requires a similar management of the cows. Game is arguably the most animal friendly meat. From the point of view of health, sensibly sourced animal proteins make a useful and valuable contribution to the human diet. Offal is the most beneficial, with a very high nutrient content. Pork can be unhealthy because of the fact that they are neither vegetarians nor fussy eaters but if raised sensibly, pork is no less healthy than other meats. Lamb, however, is healthiest even when non-organic because sheep are practically never intensively raised.

VEGETARIAN ANIMAL-BASED PROTEINS

Eggs are the best and most complete protein source for vegetarians. Like meat, eggwhite contains a record 18 amino acids, and all 10 essential amino acids, and is less likely to cause allergies than milk protein. The cholesterol in egg yolk is of no consequence to blood cholesterol. In fact, according to a study published in the British Medical Journal[2], eggs are beneficial to health and reduce cerebrovascular incidents (strokes) by 25%. Lecithin in the yolk is exceptionally high in choline (125mg per egg), a critical nutrient for acetylcholine synthesis and foetal brain development. Choline supports brain health and has been shown to slow down Alzheimer's disease and dementia. Another study also showed that choline supplementation during pregnancy can reduce the risk of the child developing schizophrenia later in life[3]. Lecithin supports cellular membrane integrity, bile production in the liver and testosterone synthesis. The dark orange yolk (the darker the better) is also rich in highly absorbable lutein, a precious antioxidant against macular degeneration. The quality of eggs depends largely on diet and the intensity of the yolk is a good indication of nutrient content in a free-range organic egg.

Quorn is a processed vegetarian protein made from a fungus-based biomass and eggwhite to bind it. It is not suitable for vegans or people with an allergy to albumin but it is also questionable in terms of immune interactions and allergic reaction. It is best avoided altogether if you have a known sensitivity to moulds, fungi or mushrooms. Even if you do not suffer from allergies you may be concerned by the battery-farmed eggwhite used in the process. Either way, I don't recommend it!

Dairy produce from cows, sheep and goats is a lesser concentrated source of vegetarian protein than eggs. Milk comes with health-related questions that are difficult to adjudicate. Depending on what you are reading, milk can be a poison

2 http://www.ncbi.nlm.nih.gov/pmc/articles/PMC3538567/
3 http://faculty.uncfsu.edu/dmontoya/About_Me_files/Journal%20of%20Neuroscience%20-%202002.pdf

unfit for human consumption or a cure for all diseases. Historically milk from various animals has certainly served man through many calamities. The argument against its components (lactose, casein, etc) being foreign to humans is simply not true as they are also found in human breast-milk.

Milk is a living product. Its virtues lie in its complicated bacterial flora which transforms milk into cheese, yoghurt, sour cream, kefir and a multitude of fermented variations. The dairy industry and its lobbies have endorsed milk pasteurisation as the only 'reliable' answer to possible contamination with pathogens like *listeria* and *E. coli*. Consequently shop-bought fermented milk products such as yoghurt have been thoroughly cooked (pasteurised) prior to fermentation. This process transforms the calcium into hard crystals and makes the milk sugar (lactose) more soluble, increasing absorption and the likelihood of blood sugar peaks that can lead to diabetes (just one of the possible health hazards associated with excessive milk consumption). Heating milk damages its fragile nutrients like vitamin C, enzymes, phosphorus and iodine. Pasteurisation may ensure that contaminated milk will not cause disease, but hygiene would surely work just as well without all the undesirable side-effects. Safety and hygiene controls are only practical on a local or small scale and impossible to implement on an industrial scale.

Raw milk and raw milk products such as butter and cheese are difficult to find, but not impossible. Sales of unpasteurised milk and cheese are banned in Scotland but can still be bought over the internet. Local farmers' markets are the simplest way to source raw milk and raw milk products that can be frozen at home. If you are not able to find raw dairy the next best thing is organic because the pasteurisation process concentrates pesticides, hormones and hormone-like milk molecules such as PCB (polychorinated biphenyl). Fermentation to produce yoghurt, fromage frais, sour cream, ghee, kefir and soft cheeses (ie feta, cottage cheese and mozzarella) improves milk digestibility. There are fewer negative reactions to raw milk and fermented dairy, but there are other considerations which may make milk unsuitable for you.

- **Casein:** casein is the main protein in milk that is concentrated in hard cheeses like Cheddar and Gruyere. It closely resembles gluten (the protein in wheat) and has been associated with similar detrimental effects on the gastro-intestinal tract lining, inflammation, allergies and auto-immune diseases. Types and concentration of casein vary depending on the animal. More traditional breeds produce milk that has lower concentrations of

BEST COOKING METHODS

Cooking at a temperature lower than 70°C conserves most of the nutrients. However higher than 110°C (steam is 100°C unless in a pressure cooker, in which case it is much hotter) destroys most of the vitamins and antioxidants like glutathione and ellagic acid. Other antioxidants and most minerals are not affected unless you are boiling the food, in which case the minerals will leach into the water. If you are making soup and consuming the water this doesn't matter, but if you are discarding the water you will be throwing away most of the nutrients. Use it for soup or stock.

Cooking isn't in itself contrary to health. In fact it sometimes greatly enhances the food by eliminating anti-nutrients, such as those found in brassicas that are damaging to the thyroid, or phytic acid found in raw nuts, seeds, grains and pulses (phytic acid is, however, eliminated by soaking as well). Cooking can even substantially increase the potency of specific antioxidants like lycopene in tomatoes.

casein and is often better tolerated by sensitive individuals. Like gluten, casein possesses opiate-like qualities that can make bread and cheese an addictive combination best kept for special occasions!

- **Lactose:** lactose, the sugar in milk, is a fermentable sugar that tends to be used up by bacteria in the fermentation process. For this reason people who are sensitive to lactose can better tolerate yoghurt, cheese, sour cream, ghee and kefir. Lactose intolerances have been associated with a deficiency in lactase, the enzyme that breaks it down and can cause inflammation of the digestive tract, diarrhoea and bloating. Lactase is often genetically deficient in people from Afro-Caribbean origins. Gut flora seems to play an important role in lactase levels and the ability to digest milk sugar. Research has shown that lactose can contribute to diabetes. Lactose should be limited and because the fat in milk slows down lactose absorption, only full fat (raw) dairy should be consumed. Avoid altogether if you have diabetic tendencies. There is no lactose in butter!

- **Milk fat:** the fat in milk is where the cow concentrates pesticides and hormones and is the main ingredient in butter – a good reason to buy only organic butter. Generally, butter and full fat dairy products have the unfounded reputation of being unhealthy because of their fat content and fat type. Health issues with milk are not linked to the type of (saturated)

Be aware, however, that grilling, browning and frying all create oxidising free radicals that are aptly called AGE (advanced glycation end-products) and known to be carcinogenic. The more you 'brown' your food, the greater the AGE content and, of course, blackened is the worst. This doesn't mean that roasted chicken can never be enjoyed but it is a good idea not to eat the skin. Similarly with roasted, grilled or barbecued food, best to leave the blackened bits on the side of your plate.

Deep-frying not only creates AGE but also damages the fat and makes it very toxic so is not recommended.

Butter, lard, coconut oil and goose fat are the most stable fats to cook with but once they start smoking they become toxic like any other heated fat. It is possible to buy phthalate-free silicone cooking pockets to use in a bain-marie. This an ideal cooking method which will preserve both flavours and nutrients.

fats found in dairy. In fact providing that it is (raw) organic, and the cows have had plenty of grass to graze on, butter is a healthy food rich in vitamins A and D and carotenoids. Additionally butter contains conjugated linoleic acid (CLA), an interesting fatty acid with positive benefits on blood sugar and diabetes that is helpful for fat-burning and to build lean muscle mass when exercising. Some researches seem to also positively point towards cholesterol and blood pressure lowering with CLA supplementation. Fermented butter is the richest in butyric acid, a valuable anti-inflammatory end product from bacterial fermentation.

- **Oestrogen and Beta-celullin:** milk naturally contains oestrogens and betacelullin, a type of growth hormone which can stimulate human growth and cancer cell proliferation. Those hormones are fat soluble and able easily to get through the intestinal wall when the milk is **homogenised.** This is because homogenisation reduces the size of the fat globules that are suspended in milk and makes it possible for them to get through un-digested and start circulating. Most milk and milk products in the market are now homogenised as well as pasteurised. Homogenisation reduces the fatty sensation of whole milk and prevents the separation of the cream. To avoid milk or dairy that has undergone homogenisation you will need to source them specifically from your local farmers' market and/or a specialist shop.

WHAT'S IN A LOAF?

In 2014 the UK bakery market was worth £3.6 billion and one of the largest sectors in the food industry. If almost 11 million loaves and packs of baked goods are sold every single day it is because their potent recipes are constructed with the sole aim of making us buy more. Processed bread and baked goods are designed to be addictive. They are packed with just the right combination of sugar, processed fats and doughy ingredients to hit the exact spot on the reward pathway of our vulnerable brain. Additionally they are stripped of most of their nutritive value, making us over fed and under-nourished, the perfect combination for cravings. As if this wasn't enough, processed bread benefits from a handy loophole that makes precise ingredients difficult to identify – because some of them can be sneaked in as processing aids.

Traditionally made sourdough bread using whole spelt or rye is far healthier than processed sliced (wholemeal) bread for a number of reasons.

Compared to modern wheat, rye and spelt contain much less gluten and amylopectin, indigestible starch elements frequently associated with

CLA naturally fixes on betacellulin receptors and neutralises most of its effect. Research remains inconclusive about the possible side-effect of dairy oestrogen. Most of it is inactive and does not show any specific correlation with breast cancer incidence. However I recommend that you reduce your dairy consumption if you have been diagnosed with an oestrogen-dependent cancer or have a family history that raises your concerns about oestrogen.

Regardless of your choice in favour or against dairy products be sure to choose organic, non-homogenised and preferably unpasteurised fermented dairy over any other form.

Goat's milk is the nearest to human breast milk and less fatty than cow's. Like ewe's and mare's, goat's milk contains less hormonal residue, is better digested, less likely to cause allergic reactions and is rarely homogenised. Goat herds tend to be smaller and bred from smaller farms with better animal welfare standards.

VEGAN PROTEINS
Vegan proteins can be found in nuts, seeds and pulses but they are of lesser

irritable bowel. Unlike yeasted bread, sourdough fermentation uses bacteria that improve the nutritional value of the flour by releasing minerals like calcium (otherwise bound with phytic acid).

Sprouted bread (Essene bread) uses grains like spelt, rye and wheat that have been sprouted first. The sprouting process radically transforms the amylopectin, thus greatly improving digestibility. Unfortunately it does not change gluten content.

Gluten-free breads are available and can be useful alternatives providing they are not overly processed or contain additives and no fibre. However, it is best to limit bread consumption to no more than 70g per day to avoid unbalancing your metabolism with excess starch. This is especially relevant if you are vegetarian and regularly consume grains and pulses as well.

Bread alternatives that contain little starch using whey protein, coconut flour and/or ground almonds are easy to make and available from the internet and some healthfood shops. They are good alternatives to bread particularly if you suffer from digestive symptoms.

quality than animal proteins. Only very few vegan proteins are complete proteins and most have to be combined in order to meet all 10 essential amino acid requirements. They are not concentrated, making protein requirements difficult to meet when following a vegan diet. This can be rectified with the addition of a protein supplement made from hemp, rice or peas. Both soya (tofu) and wheat (seitan) protein are sold as alternatives to animal proteins but I don't recommend them. Wheat protein is associated with increased allergies and soya is very frequently genetically modified, contains too many omega-6 fatty acids and frequently causes allergies. Vegan protein quality is substantially improved by soaking nuts and seeds and by sprouting pulses like chickpeas and lentils before cooking them or eating them raw. A vegan diet is also very deficient in vitamin B12 and sulphur-containing amino acids unless it includes spirulina/chlorella and plenty of seaweed. There is evidence that the B12 in blue-green algae is not absorbable and if you are following a vegan diet you should supplement with B12. Choose one that is readily absorbed and contains the activated form (methylcobalamin).

Once you have decided where you will be getting your proteins from, you will have to ensure that you are getting enough for your activity, age, metabolism, state of health and aims. One of the principal arguments against proteins is that they can be acidifying and challenging for the kidneys, especially animal proteins (muscle meat in particular) rich in sulphur amino acids (methionine and cysteine). Methionine (an essential amino-acid) is frequently blamed for its cardiovascular risk and cancer-producing metabolites. This, however, does not take into account that B12, co-existent with animal proteins together with sufficient amounts of nutrients and antioxidants effectively neutralise those acids. There is also some evidence indicating an imbalance between methionine and glycine as the cause of methionine's potential dangers. Gelatine, sesame seeds and spirulina/chlorella are rich sources of glycine.

Clearly the problem is not the proteins themselves but the balance of protein compared to essential nutrients. Also relevant is the amount your digestion can specifically handle. Eating more than 120 grams of meat at any one sitting is likely to challenge protein-digesting enzymes beyond their capacity. This leads to excessive, undigested proteins reaching the gut, feeding putrefying bacteria and releasing many cancer-promoting poisons. Here again the studies pointing to meat-eaters being more prone to bowel cancer is not an accurate evaluation of protein risks but rather a reflection of the fact that meat-eaters frequently don't care much for vegetables and eat too much at one sitting.

Because of the confusion surrounding proteins, deficiency is common especially in vegan and vegetarian diets. It leads to excess sugar and starch consumption, low energy, cravings, hunger, muscle weakness, premature ageing, saggy tissues, weight gain and lowered immunity. It is equally possible to overdo it with protein if you misleadingly believe that protein is the only food that doesn't put weight on, or if you need to have a steak on your plate before you call it a meal.

For a rough measurement of protein requirements, allow 1.8g for men (1.6g for women) of protein per kilo of body weight per day. An egg contains about 13g and 100g of steak 45g; there is 1g of protein per almond and, per dry weight, pulses are nearly 35% protein. Yoghurts and soft cheeses usually contain 7–10g of protein per 100g while hard cheeses can reach 40g. If you are struggling to reach your quota, use a protein supplement in the form of whey or, for a vegan alternative, try hemp protein.

6. LIMIT CARBOHYDRATES FROM GRAINS AND POTATOES

Grains are very rich in starch, a complex carbohydrate made up of many sugar molecules. Although this is called a 'slow' sugar and perhaps does not raise blood sugar as quickly as straightforward sugar it still has that effect. Once in the blood it will follow the same metabolic pathway as sugar. We have longer to burn it up before it turns into fat but we still have to be mindful of quantities.

Starch is made up of two specific carbohydrate molecules, amylopectin (75% –90%) and amylose (15%–20%). The proportion between those two influences the texture and the glycaemic index (the speed at which a carbohydrate will turn into blood sugar) of starchy foods. The greater the amylopectin portion the higher the glycaemic index. Depending on individual digestion, starch is more or less broken down and it is estimated that, on average, up to 20% of the starch eaten can reach the large bowel undigested where it will nourish an abundant bacterial population. Certain types of starches (in raw potatoes and green banana in particular) are even resistant to digestion altogether and referred to as 'resistant starch'.

The majority of people with digestive issues like IBS or colitis are especially ill-equipped to break down amylopectin and this can be a perpetuating factor to an already disrupted bowel flora and associated bowel inflammation. Because starches are very easily fermentable, they can contribute to a dysfunctional bowel flora by feeding the pathogen colonies. A recent study has shown that Klebsiella pneumonae possesses enzymes to thoroughly break down amylopectin and feed on it exclusively[4]. Klebsiella pneumonae in the gut is also believed to be a trigger for Crohn's disease, ulcerative colitis and ankylosing spondylitis. There is certainly plenty of empirical evidence to suggest that a low starch diet can be helpful with a variety of auto-immune diseases, inflammatory bowel diseases and even mental illness like autism.

Starchy grains (wheat, rice, rye, barley, corn, millet, buckwheat and oats) are not essential to our health or that of our probiotic population. There are sufficient carbohydrates and sugars in fresh vegetables, fruits and pulses without having to include grains and potatoes in our everyday diet. How few grains you choose to include in your diet will depend on preferences, bowel flora status, metabolic type, digestive make-up, immune function and energy requirements.

When choosing which and how much grain to eat also consider that gluten (the main protein in wheat, barley and rye) can affect gastro-intestinal permeability and contribute to bowel inflammation, auto-immune diseases and digestive discomfort. Its glue-like consistency can be a cause of constipation and by reducing grains you will also substantially limit gluten consumption. Whenever possible choose gluten-free grains like millet, buckwheat and rice. Quinoa and amaranth are great alternatives. Not technically grains as such, they are actually seeds, they are gluten-free, lower in starch than grains and a useful source of essential amino acids.

The starchy flours used habitually in baking, bread-making and batters can be partially substituted with low starch alternatives like ground almonds, bananas, grated carrots, sweet potatoes or pumpkin. Alternatively, ready-made low

---

4 http://www.hindawi.com/journals/jir/2013/872632/

carbohydrate bread, cake and pancake mixes are also available from health stores. Whey protein powder combined with ground almonds or flax and coconut flour can make a suitable alternative to grain flours for bread, muffins, pizzas and pies but will need a binding agent like eggs.

By sprouting grains you will improve their digestibility and nutritional status and reduce their starch content. Sprouted grain breads like 'Essene' breads are useful alternatives and can be bought from health food shops.

7. LIMIT FRUITS

Although fruits are packed full of antioxidants, vitamins and minerals they also contain a large amount of sugar, particularly fructose. Fructose is a direct contributor to fatty liver and closely follows the same metabolism as alcohol. Fruits should be viewed as flavouring and snacks but not as free food like vegetables. They can be incorporated into vegetable juices but a glass of fruit juice or a fruit smoothie contains so much sugar that it is no better than a chocolate bar or can of soda. The highest fructose content fruits are dried fruits, watermelon, grapes, mangoes, pears and apples. Aim to have no more than three small pieces of fresh fruit per day. For berries the equivalent of this is 200 grams.

8. CLEAN UP TOXIC CHEMICALS FROM YOUR HOME AND PERSONAL CARE

Toxic and volatile chemicals make their way into our homes through detergents, perfumes, air fresheners and even flame retardants in carpets and furniture. Some of these can be very toxic and are known to be carcinogenic. Many mimic our hormones and contribute to infertility and hormone-related symptoms. Some research has even highlighted the role of these molecules in the development of obesity and metabolic disruptions like diabetes. Ultimately they all add to our already challenged liver detoxification pathways and should be avoided as much as possible. Most are far from essential and there are many effective alternatives to wash and keep your home clean. The concept that our environment should be sterile is a commercial absurdity with absolutely no evidence of increased safety, and the impact of such products should be measured not just on our personal health but on the environment. Pollution and the degradation of our waterways, land and air concerns us all and the future of forthcoming generations.

Some common toxic chemicals in your home – and their alternatives:
- **Phthalates:** found in air fresheners and the perfumes used in detergents and conditioners. They are absorbed by the lungs and skin and are classified as hormone disrupters. They can also cause asthma and allergies. Choose

perfume-free products or those that are scented with essential oils. A few drops of lavender, lemon, orange and eucalyptus pure essential oils can be used as natural scents in cupboards and added to your steam iron water.

- **Perchlorethylene:** used as a stain remover mostly by dry-cleaners but can be found in the home. It is highly neuro-toxic and a known carcinogenic. Its usage is restricted but not banned and I suggest that you look for a dry-cleaner that specialises in avoiding toxic chemicals. Some use liquid CO_2 which is just as effective. For use in your home look for soaps and products containing ox bile to effectively remove stains.

- **Triclosan and quaternary ammonium compounds (QACs):** they are widely used as adjuncts to hygiene in domestic cleaning products. They are the active ingredients in antiseptic soaps, kitchen and bathroom sprays, laundry detergents and conditioners. They are damaging to friendly flora and serve no useful purpose. Toxic to water life and hormone disrupters, they are also implicated in antibiotic-resistant pathogens and are probable carcinogens. Some essential oils like tea-tree, lemon, birch and eucalyptus are good cleansers and can be used in liquid soap and if you need to disinfect an area. You can make your own spray cleaner using white vinegar, bicarbonate of soda and essential oils like tea tree or eucalyptus. For an alternative to laundry conditioner, a couple of tablespoons of white vinegar will eliminate static and essential oils will perfume naturally.

- **2-Butoxyethanol:** cuts through grease and is added to those 'tough' cleaners for carpets, cars, windows, ovens etc Toxic for the kidneys and a skin irritant, it is highly volatile. White vinegar mixed with bicarbonate of soda will cut through tough grease. Soda crystals are a great alternative for laundry and cleaning oily dirt and drains. Window cleaning is easy with an old newspaper and a spray bottle containing a 10% dilution of white vinegar.

- **Chlorine:** the active ingredient in bleach. Irritating for the mucous membranes in the nose and lungs, it causes allergies and its accumulation disrupts thyroid hormones and metabolisms. It is also found in tap water and swimming pools. Alternative bleaching agents using oxygen can be used and hydrogen peroxide works well against moulds in bathrooms.

- **Sodium hydroxide (caustic soda):** caustic soda is used to unblock drains and to clean ovens, but it causes burns and skin irritation. The vapours are highly toxic. Alternative drain-cleaners are highly effective and use enzymes instead. Cloths impregnated with a high concentration of diluted soda crystals, or a paste made from soda crystals, table salt and flour left overnight on encrusted grease in an oven works a treat. Steel wool will complete the action on more difficult areas.

Also present in detergent and best avoided because of reported toxicity:
Monoethanolamine (MEA)
Diethanolamine (DEA)
Triethanolamine (TEA)
Nonylphenol ethoxylates (NPE)
This is far from an exhaustive list. Unfortunately labelling is disappointingly misleading and it is not always possible to verify composition. The best policy, as with personal care products, is to use as few as possible and to keep things simple. Plain soap, white vinegar and soda crystals will sort out most cleaning issues. Essential oils are wonderfully scented and will enhance the environmental quality of any home. Some natural and effective products are available on the market to meet all laundry needs. Soap nuts are naturally soapy fruits that can be used to make the most natural and allergy-free soap and laundry detergents.

9. INCORPORATE SUPERFOODS IN YOUR DAILY DIET

Delicious, easy and packed with therapeutic nourishment: superfoods are nutrient dense foods that can be added to other foods to enhance their nutritional values. They are better than manufactured supplements because energetically in harmony with life and more readily absorbed.

- **Tart cherry juice concentrate (from Montmorency cherries)** has been shown to reduce plasma uric acid levels (a cause of gout) and to yield many positive anti-inflammatory properties[5]. They are exceptionally rich in melatonin, an anti-ageing brain hormone involved in regulating sleep quality. Take 30ml before bed to promote restorative sleep.
- **Acai berry** is known to have many anti-ageing properties because of its exceptional concentration in readily available antioxidants. It has been shown to help reduce chronic inflammation and pain[6]. improve cardiovascular health and support brain function. The best form is freeze-dried and powdered berries to maintain their fragile and quickly perishable nutritional status. It is mildly sweet and very tasty. It can be added as a sweetener to smoothies, yoghurt and deserts.
- **Organic liver** contains more bio available nutrients, gram for gram, than any other food, making them easy for your body to absorb and use.
  Liver is rich in:
  Antioxidant glutathione
  Detoxing hormone, yakriton. (May prove useful in the treatment of allergies and high histamine conditions)

---

5 http://www.fasebj.org/cgi/content/meeting_abstract/25/1_MeetingAbstracts/339.2
6 http://www.ncbi.nlm.nih.gov/pmc/articles/PMC3133683/

WHICH FRUITS CONTAIN THE MOST TOXIC CHEMICAL RESIDUES?

According to **The Environmental Working Group*** in the USA

Fruits with the least agricultural residues are those with thicker inedible skin:

1. Kiwi fruit
2. Melon
3. Pineapple
4. Citrus fruits
5. Banana (bananas are massive contributors to environmental pollution due to toxic pesticides; buy organic whenever possible)
6. Mango
7. Papaya (avoid GM papaya from Hawaii)

Fruits with the most agricultural residues:

1. Peaches and nectarines
2. Apples (more than 36 different residues!)
3. Strawberries
4. Blueberries
5. Raspberries
6. Cherries
7. Grapes
8. Pears
9. Coffee

B Vitamins, especially B12

Folic acid

Fat-soluble vitamins A, D, E and K

Essential trace elements, such as copper, zinc and selenium

Iron (liver is the best food against anaemia and is a healthier alternative to supplemental iron)

Co-enzyme Q10, crucial for heart and brain

If the idea of cooking liver regularly is just too challenging for you, it is possible to buy desiccated liver powder. Use a teaspoonful daily in water, juice, smoothie or soup. Avoid cooking desiccated liver.

- **Organic gelatine** is a versatile form of collagen. It is extracted from animal bones, skin and cartilage and is sold as gelatine or hydrolysed (liquid) collagen. It supports bone strength and joints, ligaments and skin elasticity. Traditional chicken soup and beef stock are both very rich in collagen and gelatine can be added to many sweet and savoury recipes. Another benefit of gelatine is its richness in glycine, a semi-essential amino acid involved in

---

*http://www.ewg.org/foodnews/summary.php

glucogenesis (glucose synthesis from fat in the liver), and low levels can contribute to low blood sugar. Glycine also participates actively in liver detoxification by conjugating or 'neutralising' toxic molecules such as benzoic acid (a common preservative) and is a precursor amino acid for glutathione, a major detoxification pathway in the liver. Make sure that gelatine you buy, or make from bone broth is organically sourced, as intensively raised animals can carry disease-causing prions (proteins) in their brains and in nerve tissue found in bone marrow.

- **Herbs and spices** are high in polyphenols (powerful antioxidants) which are largely responsible for their strong aromas, tastes and colours, and give them their characteristic therapeutic properties. Herbs such as oregano, thyme, rosemary and parsley; and spices such as turmeric, ginger, cinnamon, saffron and cayenne pepper have very useful health properties but also enhance food flavours. Educating our palates with a greater variety of flavours makes us more sensitive and less easily seduced by junk food such as pizzas, burgers and pastries, which are artificially engineered with taste-enhancers making them highly addictive. The complicated variety of flavours from herbs and spices breaks predictability, supports satisfaction and discourages overeating.

- **Apple cider vinegar** is a fermented food and is a useful contributor to healthy bowel flora as long as it is unpasteurised and comes with the mother (the residual material that feeds the bacteria). The specific benefits of apple cider vinegar come from its high acetic acid content which supports the function of the stomach acid. Stomach acid is frequently deficient because stress tends to suppress it and heavy foods can drain reserves. This leads to poor digestion, feeling bloated after eating, 'acid' indigestion and increased fermentation. All those symptoms can improve by taking a tablespoon of apple cider vinegar in water before meals.

  Another important function of stomach acid is its ability to control pathogenic bacteria and apple cider vinegar can support this function. This applies to the *Helicobacter pylori*, the ulcer causing bacteria that can thrive in the stomach and duodenum. Prevention is better than cure but once you have an ulcer, it is best to avoid acid and vinegar. Vinegar can be used to tenderise meat and fish, and to improve protein indigestion. It increases iron and calcium absorption. Consuming vinegar with starchy meals has been shown to increase insulin sensitivity and reduce blood sugar. When taken diluted between foods it may also help to reduce inflammation and blood triglycerides (fat) and protect arteries. This is attributed to high levels of the antioxidant chlorogenic acid[7], which has been shown to limit fat peroxidation (thought to be involved in the hardening of arteries). Preliminary research

---

7 http://www.ncbi.nlm.nih.gov/pubmed/20387813

MICROWAVE OVENS

Studies seem to point out that microwaving your food can potentially expose you to carcinogenic toxins released from plastic or paper containers. Microwaving foods also contributes to the destruction of valuable nutrients, radiation leakages and the production of radiolytic compounds. This could explain Dr Hans Hertel's controversial findings about microwaved food increasing cholesterol levels and decreasing both red and white blood cells.

Cooking or reheating in a microwave oven is best kept to a strict minimum, but if you have one in your kitchen, it can be very handy to sterilise your dishcloths, tea-towels and cleaning sponges. Those are favourable to bacterial proliferation and will harvest all sorts of undesirables. Make sure they are wet before irradiating them for a minute or so and be careful not to burn yourself when taking them out.

on rats has postulated protective properties against cardiovascular disease. Apple cider vinegar can enhance many dishes from strawberries to salad dressings. However, don't overdo it - limit consumption to 30ml a day.

- **Spirulina and chlorella** are both blue-green freshwater algae that are rich in alginate, a type of fibre with well-documented heavy metal chelation properties useful in heavy metal detoxification. It has also been shown to be radio-protective against sun radiation and radioactive compounds. Chlorella may also stimulate tissue repair and healthy tissue growth. It contains a growth factor that supports cellular DNA and slows down ageing. Look for broken cell wall chlorella to maximise its specific benefits.

Spirulina and chlorella are rich in magnesium, antioxidants and chlorophyll. and their high amino-acid content makes them both equally helpful in reducing cravings. Chlorophyll is anti-inflammatory and has been shown to have anti-cancer benefits. It's also antiseptic, stimulates healing and supports intestinal health. However, be aware that algae contain B12 analogues (false B12) that can provide false results in B12 testing and are not reliable sources of (vegan) vitamin B12. If you are a vegan ensure to get adequate amounts of B12 by taking a quality supplement daily. Methylcobalamin in a sublingual or spray form is the most readily absorbed, next to B12 injections. Check the provenance of your chlorella/spirulina by getting specific guarantees on the purity of the water and environment where they are grown. China is a major exporter of spirulina but is also renowned for its poor quality control and widespread heavy metal contamination from excessive coal-burning industries. French, Hawaiian and Australian spirulina benefit from tighter regulations and better controlled environments.

- **Sea vegetables and algae** are used extensively in Japanese foods and sushi. They spend their entire lives luxuriating in the richest, most complete mineral bath, unlike terrestrial vegetables which are limited in what they can obtain from the soil in which they grow. They soak it up and are among the best sources of iodine, magnesium, calcium, iron, zinc, potassium, manganese, and all other (56 in total) minerals essential to the human body. All this comes in perfectly absorbable form. Kelp is the most common type. In its granulated form it can be used as a salt substitute or added to bath water. Many other types of seaweeds and sea vegetables, from dulse to wakame, are worth experimenting with as condiments and snacks.

- **Whey,** along with casein is a protein found in milk. Unlike casein, which can also cause allergies, whey is high in branch chain amino acids which may help maintain lean tissue, boost fat-burning and support the immune system. Whey has been shown to have a positive effect on blood sugar in diabetics and a study published in the American Journal of Clinical Nutrition suggested it lowered levels of fat in the blood following a high-fat meal in overweight people[8]. Susan Fluegel, a nutritional biochemist at Washington State University, also found that whey protein helped lower blood pressure significantly, thus reducing the risk of stroke and heart disease[9].

  Another positive benefit of whey is its ability to increase cellular levels of glutathione (in some cases by up to 64%). Glutathione is a major free-radical scavenger and a high level in cells has been shown to protect against cancer, premature ageing and heart disease.

  Branch chain amino acids have been shown to boost muscle recovery after a workout and increase muscle strength better than other types of proteins, making whey the ideal post workout food.

  Although research doesn't make much distinction between whey protein 'isolate' and 'concentrate', it is worth bearing in mind that there are significant amounts of lactose and less protein in whey concentrate than in whey isolate. This makes whey isolate my preferred choice but only if the extraction processed is through micro-filtration and doesn't involve heat. This makes whey a very low allergy food, even for those with dairy intolerance. Whey is extremely versatile and can be used as a flour substitute in pancakes or bread, as an emulsifier in desserts, and can be easily added to yoghurt, smoothies and juices to boost their protein content.

- **Flax and Chia seeds** are exceptionally rich in alpha-linoleic acid (ALA), an

8 http://ajcn.nutrition.org/content/90/1/41.abstract?sid=81f990d4-b437-402f-be6a-10bb77c41f02
9 http://www.sciencedaily.com/releases/2010/12/101208125624.htm

omega-3 fatty acid shown to reduce inflammation and boost brain power. They are a versatile source of soluble fibre, making them invaluable for maintaining good bowel function and binding to toxins. Of the two, flax is the richest and probably the best source of the antioxidant fibres known as lignans. They have been shown to be beneficial against breast and prostate cancer and to reduce the (chronic) inflammation blood marker C-reactive protein associated with heart disease, Alzheimer's and ageing.

- **Sprouted foods:** seeds like sunflower, grains like wheat beads and pulses like chickpeas are all dormant plants waiting for the right conditions to burst into life. Germination releases the enzymes locked in these foods while substantially increasing nutritional value and eliminating anti-nutrients like phytase. Sprouting is easily done at home. Some seeds are easier to germinate than others but the process always starts by soaking them for 12 hours or so. Even if you do not wait for them to sprout fully, soaking grains, seeds and pulses prior to using them is an effective way to get rid of phytase and improve mineral absorption. **Alfalfa, fenugreek, broccoli** and **radish** make delicious salad sprouts that are especially beneficial to hormonal balance in both men and women and have been shown to be useful against breast and prostate cancer. **Aduki beans, mung beans, chickpeas** and **lentils** can be sprouted for 24 hours prior to cooking to substantially improve their digestibility and break down the oligosaccharides (galactan) responsible for their gassy nature.

- **Fermented foods** – beneficial fermentation comes from the lactic acid-producing bacteria that thrive on the sugars found in foods from milk and grains to vegetables and nuts. These bacteria play a very positive role in gut health and in supporting our own flora. There are many types of lactobacillus, the lactic acid-producing bacteria – to date 180 have been listed. Not all have been studied specifically but it's clear that types and colonies mutually support each other. It is possible to influence the type of bacteria used to ferment foods by supplementing the process with a specific shop-bought probiotic. Notable fermented products are fresh bee pollen, sauerkraut, kefir, natto, miso and yoghurt. To be beneficial they must be unpasteurised and 'live'. Once you have them you can continue to 'grow' them at home.

10. MAKE YOUR HEALTH A PRIORITY AND USE YOUR BUYING POWER WISELY

Health is not an independent experience but one that connects us to others and the environment in which we live. What we buy has consequences that may feel removed from our experience. Yet if we reduce health to a self-limited experience instead of the patient construction of our more permanent and higher self, we risk missing out on the most fundamental element of health: our core beliefs and where we see ourselves in the world. True health is not compatible with the philosophy on which consumerism is built and which states that whatever is available can be taken.

Our buying power is our greatest socio-political power. Food choices are especially relevant here. We cannot survive without food and the economic consequences are greater than with any other resources. When we eat, we participate in a transformation process that involves a chain of people which started with the growers. To be healthy, food cannot be cheap or purely functional. It has to matter and the people who contributed to it must be acknowledged. When we buy and eat consciously we are investing in **true** health.

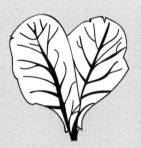

EAT YOUR
GREENS!

It is estimated that to meet her nutritional needs an average woman has to consume at least

1.25kg

OF VEGETABLES EACH DAY

in addition to a diet rich in offal, shellfish, nuts and seeds.

http://nicole.darmon.free.fr/

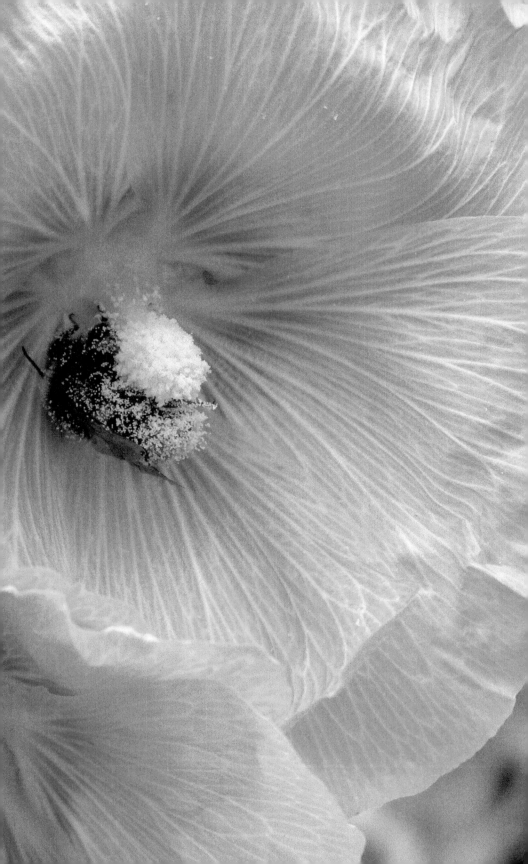

PART FIVE:
PLAN FOR YOUR
NEW LONG LIFE

"We are all here for some special reason."

ROBIN SHARMA

TIPS TO DEFY AGEING

As we have seen throughout this book defying ageing is a coordinated strategy designed to keep muscle mass high, hormones balanced, stress under control and organ function optimal. However, maintaining youthful health is an individually controlled effort because we all have our own specific physical and mental make-up which makes us more or less resilient to the challenges of time and life.

The following are my top five tips for age-defying health management:

1. IDENTIFY YOUR PHYSIOLOGICAL WEAKNESSES AND PACE YOURSELF

Some of us put on weight easily, others don't; we might have a weak digestion, a susceptibility to colds or a skin that blemishes at the first signs of stress. Deadlines might motivate us or make us feel tense and anxious, sleep might be difficult or something we can quickly fall into whenever we need a rest.

Whatever your particular personality and specific physiology, learn to pay attention and to recognise your weaknesses, as well as your strengths in order to pace yourself accordingly.

2. IDENTIFY WHAT MAKES YOU FEEL NOTICEABLY WORSE AND AVOID IT

We are far from equal when it comes to metabolising alcohol, caffeine, additives, drugs and medication. Know your body and recognise how much you are affected by them. The old adage that an occasional take-away or a glass of wine won't harm you may be true for some but not necessarily for you.

Similarly our sensitivity to sugar varies greatly. The smallest amount of processed sugary foods may be a trigger for uncontrollable cravings and a contributor to anxiety and stress, or you might find that a dessert eaten with friends or family is a way to share and connect with little or no other consequence.

Digestion is perhaps a direct and immediate barometer to assess your body's response to certain foods or drinks, but fatigue, mood swings, restless sleep, aches and pains, brain fog, dryness, thirst and itchiness are all symptoms of toxic build-up and the need for avoiding the worst offenders.

Be aware that lack of sleep, inactivity, emotional stress and environmental quality are factors which are equally, if not more, important to health and ageing than what you put in your mouth.

Be aware and honestly look for connections regardless of what others might say. It is your body and only you know how you feel at any given time and what you are sensitive to.

3. IDENTIFY THE STRATEGIES THAT CAN QUICKLY MAKE YOU FEEL BETTER AND ALLOW TIME FOR THEM

Depending on your personality type you might find that a massage will ground you when you are feeling stressed or that a session at the gym does the job better. You might be able to sleep 12 hours straight and wake up refreshed or prefer a 30-minute nap in the middle of the day to compensate for less than optimal sleep. A sauna might help lift brain fog and a long swim wash away anxiety. Avoiding alcohol for a couple of weeks could help you to refocus and reinforce your willpower, or doing a day of vegetable juices might achieve greater wellbeing in a very short time. Sometimes we need to talk to friends and get perspective; sometimes we need to spend a day being quiet and reflect. Know what works for you and put it in your diary to make sure that you regularly cultivate wellness.

4. LEARN TO ASK FOR HELP AND SUPPORT

Asking for help is not the same as sharing frustration or expressing distress. Although off-loading can feel helpful it is short-lived. To ask for help means we don't have to do it alone and we have to formulate and clarify what we need in order to involve someone else. It is not a sign of weakness and we all need help at some time. Asking for help doesn't have to be about your health to benefit your health; just to feel supported is enough.

5. PRACTISE GRATITUDE

Gratitude is a kind of empathetic mindfulness which keeps us connected to others and maintains a positive mental attitude. It is good for our health, with plenty of evidence to support this, and, unlike love which is a state or a feeling, gratitude can be practised and developed. What's more, it can be practised any time and whatever the circumstances. Indeed you will notice that as well as your friends and family, lots of people are participating in and contributing to your life, from those who grow your food to those who maintain your surroundings, drive the trains you travel on and serve you in shops. A beggar on a street corner can even be an opportunity to practise gratitude for the chance to be charitable!

STRATEGIES TO GET YOU THROUGH

When it comes to dietary commitment, success is 15% willpower and 85% preparation. By planning ahead and by developing useful supportive strategies you will be able to enjoy all the fun or face the demands of a busy life without losing your focus or spending longer than necessary on it.

The relationship the French have with food has inspired much research and writing. In 2010 the French gastronomic meal, and every activity connected with the event including the shopping and preparation, was listed by UNESCO as an Intangible Cultural Heritage of Humanity.

Compared to other countries, French women have a reputation for staying slim despite their penchant for patisseries and French men for resisting cardiovascular disease while enjoying red wine. This surprising ability even has a name 'the French paradox'. It has been scientifically studied and has been much written about.

I was brought up in the French tradition; my mother went to the top hotel and catering school. Before that and during World War II my grandfather kept a restaurant. During the day my grandmother would prepare inventive dishes made from wild food caught or picked locally, while at night my grandfather was in the woods fighting in the Resistance.

Clichés about the French and their obsessions with food attempt to highlight one magic element, but fail to identify the simple lessons we can all take from a nation that has made food a way of life. It is not that French women don't get fat when they eat pastries or that French men have a special alcohol-resistant gene. It is more that the French are mindful about eating and, consequently, the experience of eating and sharing food becomes a fulfilling experience. They are selective about the company they keep at mealtimes and inquisitive about what they put in their mouth. They carefully plan their meal, walk that extra mile or are willing to pay more for a product that's been prepared locally rather than industrially. They will readily fast by skipping a meal or two in order to enjoy a special occasion among friends.

Slow, shared, planned and mindful eating achieves one thing above all and that's portion control. When it comes to health this is fundamental. Too much food (even healthy food) or alcohol is never a good idea no matter the circumstance!

THE FOLLOWING ARE STRATEGIES AIMED AT PORTION CONTROL:

- **Start a meal with soup or fresh vegetable juice:** This is backed up by observational studies. Take your time and let the appetite hormones regulate for what follows. The more flavoursome, the more it will stimulate pleasure receptors and induce satisfaction.
- **Make a point to have less than you want and wait before taking more:** 20 minutes makes all the difference between feeling satisfied and feeling hungry. Even if you want seconds you are more likely to have less and enjoy it more after a 15 to 20-minute interval.
- **Eat a protein snack before going out to a dinner or a party:** It's always easier to control quantity when not hungry. Never go to a dinner party feeling hungry. Proteins stave off hunger without filling you up. A plain yoghurt with whey protein, a boiled egg or lean chicken are all possibilities.
- **Never drink alcohol on an empty stomach:** This has repeatedly been proven to reduce self-control!
- **Stay away from the salty snacks at parties:** Once you start you won't be able to stop. This is not a myth, thanks to carefully engineered and top secret recipes. It is no coincidence that the exact ingredients are top secret. The same goes for sodas. Sparkling water with a slice of orange, lemon or lime keeps your mind and palate busy. I like to add fresh mint, fennel or rosemary leaves. If you want an alcoholic drink choose one with minimal sugar content like gin or vodka. You can also add Angostura bitters to your sparkling water. This will stimulate your liver and digestive enzymes and support digestion.
- **Desserts is stressed spelt backwards:** This should speak for itself if you can remember it at the appropriate time. If you forget then at least remember that a flourless chocolate cake is likely to be smaller, less sugary and gluten-free and therefore preferable to a *tarte Tatin* with icecream and caramel sauce; in other words, don't be fooled by the apples, look for something small. Sorbets are gentle on the palate and the least costly on your waistline. How we feel about the dessertson offer has a lot to do with how we imagine them. When we look at a menu we build a perception of what each item is and how delicious we might find it. Visualise each dish, imagine how sweet, heavy and dense it is and then hand the menu back to the waiter saying: "Lovely, but no thanks".
- **Lack of sleep** contributes to sugar, carb and alcohol cravings: regularly sleeping less than six hours disrupts appetite hormones and growth hormone, leading to insulin resistance. Together these factors make portion control harder and induce craving. Make a point to have early nights regularly and to sleep longer. This also improves work efficiency and clarity of mind.

THE 7-DAY BACK-TO-HEALTH EATING PLAN

The dietary planners are to help you apply the principles of choice in a constructive way depending on your taste preferences.
Choose the detox option:

TO LOSE WEIGHT

The most efficient way to lose weight is to alternate detox days with non-detox days (see the Detox Planners on the following seven pages). Follow for as long as you need to reach your target weight. The idea is not to restrict your overall calorie intake, but to briefly and regularly put your body into food shortage mode which forces it to burn stored fat. This will also improve metabolic rate, regulate hormone balance and keep cells vibrant – all fundamental requirements for anti-ageing and lasting good health. Exercise is especially useful and can be done on detox days for an additional metabolic boost.

TO RECOVER AFTER A PERIOD OF EXCESS OR IF FEELING LOW

Follow the detox days for three to seven days depending on time available. Combine with sauna, colonic hydrotherapy and exercise to stimulate detox. If you are generally healthy even as little as three days will yield remarkable benefits.

TO IMPROVE ENERGY LEVELS, STIMULATE THE IMMUNE SYSTEM AND RECOVER FROM ILLNESS OR SURGERY

Aim to follow the **non-vegetarian** options for six days and the detox options for one day each week. In most cases people will start to improve after two to three weeks. This is a profound lifestyle shift, however, and not a quick fix. Depending on your health you may need the support of a naturopathic practitioner and to consider more specific dietary elements. However this is a very good place to start. If you cannot bring yourself to eat meat switch to the vegetarian options.

TO ADDRESS CHRONIC ILLNESS AND REDUCE INFLAMMATION

Follow the **non-vegetarian** options until you feel noticeably better; then start to introduce the detox days once per week if you are underweight or twice a week if not. Seek professional support to assist you and explore more specific dietary elements. If you cannot bring yourself to eat meat switch to the vegetarian options but do not eat any dairy except for butter and whey protein isolate (practically lactose free).

DAY 1	BREAKFAST	LUNCH	DINNER	SNACK	DRINKS
Super-detox	Chia pudding: soak overnight ½ cup of chia seeds in coconut milk or water **Flavour** with cinnamon, walnuts and a grated apple	A very large raw vegetable and avocado salad **Season** with olive oil, apple cider vinegar and roasted pumpkin seeds	Whey protein smoothie with ground flax. Add water to the desired consistency **Mix** with spinach, avocado and mango	Vegetable juice of your choice. Limit fruits to no more than ⅓ **Try** beetroot and orange	Green tea Herbal tea (not fruity because often artificially flavoured) 1 or 2 cups black coffee (optional)
Vegetarian	2 eggs, thyme and mushroom omelette cooked in coconut butter	Lentils and orange salad seasoned with olive oil, balsamic vinegar and oregano	A roasted sweet potato and hummus served with a mixed salad	2 slices of carb-free bread (see Basic Recipes) spread with feta cheese	**Optional drinks:** • A small glass of wine • 1 cup hot chocolate made from cacao and almond milk or water, sweetened with dried lucuma powder (a type of fruit) or stevia. For additional creaminess add coconut butter • 1 or 2 cups black coffee or tea. Coconut butter can be used as a milk substitute • Bone broth (See Recipes) consommé once or twice daily
Non-vegetarian	Vegetable juice of your choice	Avocado and cucumber sandwich made from carb-free bread (see Basic Recipes) served with a mixed salad	Roast chicken and vegetables cooked in coconut butter and seasoned with mixed herbs (oregano, thyme rosemary and sage)	Plain bio yoghurt with ground flax (available from health stores), whey protein and berries	
In a hurry	½ cup of soaked chia seeds with plain bio - yoghurt, whey protein, nuts and a piece of fresh fruit or berries of your choice	Shop-bought roast chicken breast and cherry tomatoes	Gluten-free wrap (see Basic Recipes) with feta cheese and a mixed salad	Avocado with 100% rye crackers	

DAY 2	BREAKFAST	LUNCH	DINNER	SNACK	DRINKS
Super-detox	Chia pudding: soak overnight ½ cup of chia seeds in coconut milk or water **Flavour** with raw cacao powder	A very large raw vegetable and avocado salad **Season** with walnut oil, apple cider vinegar and roasted pine nuts	Whey protein smoothie with ground flax. Add water to the desired consistency **Mix** with banana, spirulina and raw cacao powder	Vegetable juice of your choice. Limit fruits to no more than ⅓ **Try** orange, carrot and coriander	Green tea Herbal tea (not fruity because often artificially flavoured) 1 or 2 cups black coffee (optional)
Vegetarian	Vegetable juice of your choice	Baby spinach and raspberry salad served with roasted pine nuts and 2 boiled eggs, olive oil and apple cider vinegar dressing	Roasted sweet peppers filled with feta and quinoa and served with a mixed salad of your choice	Almond butter on 2 slices of carb-free bread (see Basic Recipes)	**Optional drinks:** • A small glass of wine • 1 cup hot chocolate made from cacao and almond milk or water, sweetened with dried lucuma powder (a type of fruit) or stevia. For additional creaminess add coconut butter
Non-vegetarian	Plain bio yoghurt with ground flax (from health store), whey protein with a piece of fresh fruit or berries of your choice	Chicken breast, dried tomatoes and Parmesan with baby leaf salad seasoned with olive oil and balsamic vinegar	Quinoa and feta tabouli made with fresh chopped mint, diced tomatoes, olive oil, lemon juice and roasted pine nuts	Banana loaf (see Recipes)	• 1 or 2 cups black coffee or tea. Coconut butter can be used as a milk substitute • Bone broth (see Recipes) consommé once or twice daily
In a hurry	2 boiled eggs and sprouted wheat bread (from health store)	Tomato, avocado and mozzarella salad with olive oil and fresh basil	Chicken breast and steamed vegetables of your choice	Plain bio yoghurt with ground flax (from health store), whey protein with a piece of fresh fruit or berries of your choice	

DAY 3	BREAKFAST	LUNCH	DINNER	SNACK	DRINKS
Super-detox	Chia pudding: soak overnight ½ cup of chia seeds in coconut milk or water **Flavour** with vanilla	A very large raw vegetable and avocado salad **Season** with lemon juice and olive oil	Whey protein smoothie with ground flax. Add water to the desired consistency: **Mix** with cucumber, fresh mint and lime	Vegetable juice of your choice. Limit fruits to no more than ⅓ **Try** red peppers, tomatoes and celery	Green tea Herbal tea (not fruity because often artificially flavoured) 1 or 2 cups black coffee (optional)
Vegetarian	Almond butter on 2 slices of carb-free bread (see Basic Recipes)	Scrambled eggs and tomatoes cooked in coconut butter served with a mixed salad	Lentil burger made by mixing ½ cup of sprouted lentils with ½ cup of grated courgettes, 2 tablespoons tahini, 2 tablespoons ground flax and 1 egg. Season with spring onions, herbs etc Let it stand 15 minutes before lightly cooking in coconut oil	Plain bio yoghurt with ground flax (from health store), whey protein and berries	**Optional drinks:** • A small glass of wine • 1 cup hot chocolate made from cacao and almond milk or water, sweetened with dried lucuma powder (a type of fruit) or stevia. For additional creaminess add coconut butter • 1 or 2 cups black coffee or tea. Coconut butter can be used as a milk substitute • Bone broth (see Recipes) consommé once or twice daily
Non-vegetarian	Smoked salmon served with cucumber and sour cream on a slice of carb-free bread (see Basic Recipes) or gluten-free oatcakes	Quinoa, grated cucumber and roasted pine nut salad. Season with olive oil and lemon juice		Vegetable juice of your choice. Limit fruits to no more than ⅓ **Try** red peppers, tomatoes and celery	
In a hurry	Tahini on sprouted wheat bread (from health store)	Tinned tuna fish served with diced cucumber in a yoghurt and olive oil dressing seasoned with dill	Steamed vegetables, sun-dried tomatoes and feta cheese medley. **Flavour** with turmeric and coconut butter	Vegetable juice of your choice. Limit fruits to no more than ⅓ Try red peppers, tomatoes and celery	

DAY 4	BREAKFAST	LUNCH	DINNER	SNACK	DRINKS
Super-detox	Chia pudding: soak overnight ½ cup of chia seeds in coconut milk or water **Flavour** with rose water, lucuma powder (from health store) and roasted chopped pistachios	A very large raw vegetable and avocado salad **Season** with sun-dried tomatoes, olive oil, and gomasio (roasted sesame salt available from health stores)	Whey protein smoothie with ground flax. Add water to the desired consistency **Mix** with peach, fresh mint and lamb's lettuce	Vegetable juice of your choice. Limit fruits to no more than ¹/₃ **Try** cucumber, mint and lime	Green tea Herbal tea (not fruity because often artificially flavoured) 1 or 2 cups black coffee (optional)
Vegetarian	Banana pancakes made by blending a ripe medium size banana and an egg with a pinch of salt. Lightly fry in coconut butter	Grated carrots and coriander salad served with hummus	Steamed vegetable, sun-dried tomato, olive oil and feta cheese medley. **Season** with herbs	A smoothie made from 2 tablespoons whey protein, ¼ of pineapple and 1 tablespoon coconut butter. Add water to the desired consistency	**Optional drinks:** • 1 small glass wine • 1 cup hot chocolate made from cacao and almond milk or water; sweetened with dried lucuma powder (a type of fruit) or stevia. For additional creaminess add coconut butter
Non-vegetarian	A ripe banana spread on 2 slices of carb-free bread (see Basic Recipes)	Sprouted lentil and orange salad served with rocket and roasted pumpkin seeds. **Season** with pumpkin oil, balsamic vinegar and ground turmeric	Lambs' liver cooked in coconut oil turmeric served with onion marmalade and seasonal vegetables	Plain bio yoghurt, cashew nuts, whey protein and chopped banana flavoured with cacao powder	• 1 or 2 cups black coffee or tea. Coconut butter can be used as a milk substitute]
In a hurry	½ cup of soaked chia seeds with plain bio yoghurt, whey protein, nuts and a piece of fresh fruit or berries of your choice	Scrambled eggs and spring onions cooked in coconut butter	Chicken breast and steamed vegetables	2 slices of sprouted wheat bread (from health store) with almond butter	• Bone broth consommé once or twice daily

DAY 5	BREAKFAST	LUNCH	DINNER	SNACK	DRINKS
Super-detox	Chia pudding: soak overnight ½ cup of chia seeds in coconut milk or water **Flavour** with blueberries and grated coconut	A very large raw vegetable and avocado salad **Season** with olives, olive oil, lemon juice and oregano	Whey protein smoothie with ground flax. Add water to the desired consistency **Mix** with kale cacao spirulina and banana	Vegetable juice of your choice. Limit fruits to no more than ¹/₃ **Try** carrots, ginger, orange and fresh coriander	Green tea Herbal tea (not fruity because often artificially flavoured) 1 or 2 cups black coffee (optional)
Vegetarian	Raspberry, cacao and whey protein smoothie made with almond milk	Vegetable soup and carb-free bread (see basic recipes)	Courgette patty: Mix ½ cup of mashed courgette or pumpkin, 2 tablespoons of ground flax and an egg season and lightly fry in coconut butter. Serve with a mixed salad	Oat bran and pumpkin muffin (see Recipes)	**Optional drinks:** • 1 small glass wine • 1 cup hot chocolate made from cacao and almond milk or water, sweetened with dried lucuma powder (a type of fruit) or stevia. Add coconut butter for creaminess • 1 or 2 cups black coffee or tea. Coconut butter can be used as a milk substitute • Bone broth consommé once or twice daily
Non-vegetarian	Banana loaf (see Recipes)	Smoked salmon served with diced cucumber in walnut oil and yoghurt dressing seasoned with turmeric and dill	Turkey burger made by mixing 100g ground turkey meat with 2 tablespoons ground flax and 1 egg. Add a little water and stand for 15 minutes before shallow-frying in coconut butter	Chocolate mousse made by blending avocado with mango and cacao powder	
In a hurry	Plain bio yoghurt cashew nuts, whey protein and chopped banana flavoured with cacao powder	Chicken and vegetable soup (see Basic Recipes) with 100% rye bread This can be made in advance and frozen	Tuna steak served with capers and a mixed salad of your choice	½ an avocado seasoned with lemon juice	

DAY 6	BREAKFAST	LUNCH	DINNER	SNACK	DRINKS
Super-detox	Chia pudding: soak overnight ½ cup of chia seeds in coconut milk or water **Flavour** with ground almonds and pear	A very large raw vegetable and avocado salad **Season** with chopped pecan nuts and fresh figs	Whey protein smoothie with ground flax. Add water to the desired consistency **Mix** with parsley, cucumber and ¼ pineapple	Vegetable juice of your choice. Limit fruits to no more than ⅓ **Try** fennel, carrots and lemon	Green tea Herbal tea (not fruity because often artificially flavoured) 1 or 2 cups black coffee (optional)
Vegetarian	Banana, spirulina, cacao and whey protein smoothie made with almond milk	Fennel, chopped orange and sesame seed salad served with millet or quinoa	Roasted butternut squash and goat's cheese served with a salad of your choice	Carb-free bread (see Basic Recipes) spread with almond butter	**Optional drinks:** • 1 small glass wine • 1 cup hot chocolate made from cacao and almond milk or water, sweetened with dried lucuma powder (a type of fruit) or stevia. For additional creaminess add coconut butter
Non-vegetarian	Banana, spirulina, cacao and whey protein smoothie made with almond milk	A large salad with avocado, olives and feta cheese	Chicken and vegetable curry made with coconut cream served with millet or quinoa	Banana loaf (see Recipes)	• 1 or 2 cups black coffee or tea. Coconut butter can be used as a milk substitute
In a hurry	A ripe banana on 2 slices of 100% rye bread spread with almond butter	Avocado, tomato, olives and feta salad seasoned with oregano, olive oil and balsamic vinegar dressing	2 scrambled eggs served with smoked salmon and a mixed salad	30g very dark chocolate (min 85%) and 10 walnuts	• Bone broth consommé once or twice daily

DAY 7	BREAKFAST	LUNCH	DINNER	SNACK	DRINKS
Super-detox	Chia pudding: soak overnight ½ cup of chia seeds in coconut milk or water **Flavour** with orange blossom water, ground cardamom and papaya	A very large raw vegetable and avocado salad **Season** with mixed sunflower, sesame and pumpkin seeds	Whey protein smoothie with ground flax. Add water to the desired consistency. **Mix** with rocket and mandarin	Vegetable juice of your choice. Limit fruits to no more than ¹/₃ **Try** sweet potato, cucumber, lime and ginger	Green tea Herbal tea (not fruity because often artificially flavoured) 1 or 2 cups black coffee (optional)
Vegetarian	Arrow root gluten-free wrap (see Basic Recipes) served with berries and yoghurt	Grilled halloumi cheese skewer served with a grilled butternut and rocket salad seasoned with a sesame oil and vinegar dressing	Sprouted chick peas and vegetable curry made with coconut cream and served with quinoa	Very dark chocolate (min 85%) and 10 walnuts	**Optional drinks:** • 1 small glass wine • 1 cup hot chocolate made from cacao and almond milk or water, sweeten edwith dried lucuma powder (a type of fruit) or stevia. For additional creaminess add coconut butter • 1 or 2 black coffee or tea. Coconut butter can be used as a milk substitute • Bone broth consommé, a mug fuldaily
Non-vegetarian	Plain bio yoghurt cashew nuts, whey protein and a grated apple with cinnamon	Avocado, dried tomato, anchovy, olive and Parmesan salad seasoned with oregano, olive oil and balsamic vinegar dressing	Grilled tuna steak served with tomato, onions and squash ratatouille seasoned with mixed herbs	Oat bran and pumpkin muffin(see Basic Recipes)	
In a hurry	A ripe banana on 2 slices of 100% rye bread spread with almond butter	Boiled eggs and steamed asparagus	Grilled liver and cauliflower mash mixed with butter and 2 tablespoons ground flax. Season to taste and stand for 10 minutes before eating	Hummus and vegetable sticks	

PUTTING IT INTO PRACTICE

The following are stories from some of my clients. I have picked them because they illustrate how better health is more about changing a mindset than about following a protocol. They illustrate the importance of putting each person into a physical, emotional and biochemical context and of coordinating change between realistic expectations and effective methods. All gave their permission but some asked me to change their names.

EMILY'S STORY
WEIGHT GAIN, A SURPRISING CONSEQUENCE
OF UNDERLYING GLUTEN SENSITIVITY

Emily, like so many women in their fifties, came to see me because she was constipated. She felt sluggish and bloated and blamed her menopause for the loss of energy and listlessness that had gradually taken over her life. She had already tried most of my usual recommendations for better evacuation and none were producing much result. In fact taking laxatives was all she could do to open her bowels. Emily was gaining weight, craved sugar and generally felt disconnected with herself. Her grown-up daughter, she told me, suffered from an auto-immune thyroid disease. Emily had a happy relationship which only compounded her sense of inadequacy for not feeling more enthusiastic about it. She was particularly fond of wine gums and carried a bag with her wherever she went. Hers were naturally flavoured because she paid attention to her food which she generally cooked from scratch, and included plenty of fresh fruit and vegetables.

When I explained to Emily that her thyroid was playing a big part in her weight gain, constipation and low mood she wasn't surprised, having witnessed her daughter's difficulties. She was surprised to hear that gluten, food allergies and sugar all conspired to low grade widespread inflammation in her body and contributed to her metabolism slowing down. I suggested she stop eating foods with gluten, including the wine gums which also contain gluten as well as sugar.

This helped her constipation and she felt a little better for opening her bowels more regularly. On each of Emily's monthly visits to me she would report on the various reasons she had to come off her diet: an important gluten-rich party at one of her husband's wealthy clients or a gluten-packed holiday in France or Italy. This actually went on for almost nine months. Emily was fairly convinced that the gluten was not good for her but she couldn't connect it to her general state. It took three separate incidents to create the prefect storm and finally get her to understand that she had to commit to her health before it could improve. First she discovered that her husband was having an affair, then, a week later, she blacked out and woke up on the kitchen floor with blood on her face. As a result she was prescribed blood tests by her doctor which revealed that she was borderline diabetic, severely anaemic, and that she had too much cholesterol. He told her to cut down on fat and sugar and to take an iron supplement even if constipation was a certain side effect. That's when I saw her again, she was ready to put herself first and take control of her health. No one was going to do it for her.

This time I asked Emily to keep a food diary and write down everything she ate and drank and how she felt for seven days. When she came back we analysed everything and got her started on whey protein and superfoods smoothies every morning to help control her sugar cravings and boost her antioxidants. We made sure that she threw out all the remaining wine gums, gluten and processed foods that were still lurking in her kitchen cupboards and she started to see a personal trainer at a local gym twice weekly. This was the beginning of a transformation that lasted almost a year and saw Emily regain confidence, fitness and health. As a result she decided to enrol on a counselling course and is now enjoying a full and active life.

FRANK'S STORY
DEPRESSION CAN SIMPLY BE A SIGN
OF A STRESSED AND TIRED NERVOUS SYSTEM

Frank was in his mid-fifties when he came to see me. His wife had told him that before throwing in the towel and quitting his business, he should come and speak to me. Frank looked grey, tired and overweight but what struck me about him was that he couldn't sit still; his right leg was constantly moving up and down, his breathing was fast and shallow, his jaw was tightening and relaxing and he kept shifting position on his seat. This was someone who felt profoundly uncomfortable in his own body, but why? He did not lack confidence and he had achieved great things. Family life was stable and business performance was still successful despite his declining involvement with it. He was ready to retire but had no idea what he was going to do instead. All he could say was that he was bored and couldn't see the point. Money was not an issue and nothing really got him excited. Listening to Frank it would have been easy to say that he was mildly depressed and his doctor had alluded to antidepressants, but on closer inspection it became apparent that Frank was stressed. His body couldn't let go; he was not getting any meaningful sleep or restorative downtime. When I asked about his diet and lifestyle, he was having sugary coffee every two hours and half a bottle of wine most evenings. He ate out a lot but never ordered desserts. He craved strong savoury foods like mature cheeses and anchovies which he brought back from his numerous business trips to Italy. Frank had really agreed to see me only at his wife's request and I was finding it difficult to establish how I could help him. He wasn't sleeping well and this did bother him but before I could mention coffee or wine I had to get him a little more interested. I asked him to think of a moment in his life when he enjoyed a profound sense of accomplishment and felt valued and purposeful, something that he remembered as a special time. He told me about his experience as a university student when he had been a member of a choir for four years.

Every year they held concerts in a nearby country house. This was always a bit of an event because the host put on a garden party to which it was a great honour to be invited. The choir concert was the highlight of the afternoon and every year was a challenge to surpass the previous year's performance. There were only 18 choir members and the lead-up to the event made everyone bond very strongly. There was no competition; all played their part and all felt the same contagious excitement about the event.

I got Frank to tell me about those four occasions. The music they chose, the weather on the day, the variations in the group as some of the members completed their degrees and moved on. For 20 minutes I saw Frank's face light up with excitement at the thought of those special moments. I knew that if I could convince him to join a choir and sing again he would have to breathe more deeply and the rest would follow. It took some convincing and he made a couple of attempts before finding a choir that would accept him but the night after his first practice he slept better than he had in years. His wife called me to tell me. She also told me that during the four weeks it took Frank to get himself organised with the choir he hadn't once mentioned retiring and seemed a lot less irritable. I was invited to the Christmas carol concert the following year. Frank's complexion was rosier and he had lost a little weight (or perhaps it was just his posture that was better) but mostly he was smiling and I recognised the sparkle in his eyes which I had briefly witnessed the previous year.

AHMED'S STORY
A FATTY LIVER DOESN'T ALWAYS COME FROM ALCOHOL

Ahmed came to see me because he had been diagnosed with the beginnings of a fatty liver. His doctor was concerned about the fact, that at 34, he was too young to be heading for liver disease and had lectured him on alcohol intake. Ahmed was very confused because he had no symptoms (this is typical of a fatty liver), he didn't drink alcohol for religious reasons, went to the gym every day and looked strong and fit.

Ahmed had done his own research on the internet and knew that fructose was a cause of non-alcoholic fatty liver. As a result he was very careful about his fruit consumption but did not quite realise that fructose was also in the energy drinks that he consumed during his daily workout and in the regular sugar he was adding to his tea and porridge in the morning.

He also consumed daily protein drinks that contained sucralose, an artificial sugar clinically proven to negatively alter gut flora and to interfere with liver enzymes. He ate a lot of dairy products because he thought that those counted as protein and he was restricting carbohydrates to help with his body-building efforts at the gym.

I began by alerting Ahmed to the convincing evidence that altered gut flora is a big contributor to liver disease. I also explained to him about the sugar (lactose) in milk which is made up of one molecule of glucose and one molecule of galactose. In the liver, galactose has an identical pathway to fructose and alcohol and will directly contribute to fatty liver.

Together we agreed that he had to change his protein shake recipe and stop dairy and energy drinks. We replaced cow's milk with almond and coconut milk and started to make his protein shakes from pure whey isolate to which he added plant-based antioxidants, a probiotic blend and extra omega-3 fatty acids. I told him to use fresh fruits (especially berries) to sweeten the shakes.

I recommended him to eat organic liver twice weekly and, if this was difficult, to use desiccated liver instead. None of this seemed particularly difficult for him to do and he embraced it all very positively. I asked him to book an appointment with his doctor three months later and to call me to rearrange an appointment once he had the test results.

He did call me but together we decided that a follow-up appointment was not necessary. He was feeling great; all the liver function tests had come back negative. He was just happy to continue on his new health routine.

JULIE'S STORY
CHRONIC FATIGUE: SOMETIMES LESS IS MORE

Julie came to see me as part of her long and slow recovery from chronic fatigue. Her condition had been particularly debilitating and her symptoms, although much improved, were still controlling most of her day. She had to meticulously plan various tasks, like doing the laundry, because she knew that it would leave her exhausted and give her severe and lasting muscle pain. Her arms and upper back were the worst. She couldn't tell me how it all started but a traumatic break-up six years previously combined with her mother's sudden death had precipitated matters. I learned that, as a child, Julie had been sickly and taken lots of antibiotics. As an infant she could not keep her milk down and was prescribed Milk of Magnesia.

More recently she had suffered from a tooth abscess that had penetrated the gum and required two months of antibiotics. Julie had already consulted different practitioners and was on a very controlled diet. She avoided grains, dairy, alcohol and sugar and took numerous supplements, from herbal supports to anti-oxidants and probiotics. There wasn't much she hadn't covered nutritionally and she was seeking my advice to learn more about detox. I explained to her that detox was a continuous process consisting in breaking down and neutralising the various toxic molecules that found their way into our blood. When this wasn't possible, for whatever reasons, a toxic molecule could also be sequestered into fatty tissues.

However, detox is only half the story, the other half is elimination. Without efficient elimination all the detoxed metabolites (the remaining bits) would be left in the liver ducts, bowel and kidneys and could be reconstructed back into their original toxic forms, especially if bowel bacteria were off kilter and up for the job. Indeed her past antibiotic use had most certainly weakened her gut flora and the bacteria were adding to the toxic burden.

I suggested that Julie commit to weekly colonic hydrotherapy and combined her treatments with (green) vegetable juices and bone broth fasting. Gall bladder flushing was planned to take place every four or six weeks depending on her response to the protocol.

She always seemed to be better for not eating and the gall bladder flushing was thankfully never that challenging to her. I always recommend a colonic irrigation after a gall bladder flush. It helps with the elimination from the liver and gall bladder, and what is actually released is made up of bile, gall stones and cholesterol crystals. Because I can see what is released (through clear tubes) I can also appraise how productive a flush has been. In Julie's case the first three were reasonable but the fourth one was truly spectacular and left her feeling euphoric for the first time in years. It also motivated her to continue with her treatment protocol for nine consecutive months; each time positive gains were made and Julie is now much improved. She turned a corner following that fourth flush and to this day continues with regular flushing and juice fasting.

STUART'S STORY
IS ADDICTION JUST A SYMPTOM?

Stuart is a gay writer. Not that this should matter but that's how he first introduced himself to me: "Hello, I'm Stuart and I'm a gay writer." At the time I wasn't sure if he was referring to his sexual orientation or his jovial nature because he was both camp and very energetic…but Stuart had a secret: he was addicted to painkillers, tramadol to be precise. This made him terribly constipated. It had all started after a car accident where he had suffered whiplash and a broken wrist. At the time he thought nothing of it but four years down the line he could not get out of bed without it. Every morning his happy nature was submerged by the blackest cloud until he took his first tramadol with lots of strong coffee. Shortly after that his life was bright again. For him, taking his painkillers was like opening the curtains and letting the sun stream in.

Because his main problem was constipation I had to focus on his bowel. I made all the usual recommendations about ground omega-3-rich flax seeds, a high-fibre diet with increased fluid intake. I suggested he used lecithin to improve liver function and provide additional lubrication, as well as a strong bio-magnesium supplement. I also told him to take regular Epsom salt baths to increase the magnesium and the sulphur in his body and to support good (drug) detoxification. I explained to Stuart how magnesium served many purpose in terms of bowel health and detoxification but it can also enhance the effects of opiates. I encouraged him to experiment with dosages and timing. To further stimulate his bowel I recommended that he use spicy foods especially black pepper, cayenne pepper and turmeric because they have been shown to have marginal analgesic benefits. Black pepper also contains an active ingredient, piperine, which greatly improves the delivery of certain molecule including opiates. Here again Stuart was to experiment with reducing his painkillers on the basis that effects were enhanced.

When I saw Stuart six weeks later he had made good progress and had reduced his painkillers. He had got himself into a routine about bowel movements and supplement intake and he was developing a taste for hot foods. I was thrilled to hear that he had spoken to his doctor about his addiction and they were working together for Stuart to gradually come off the drug. I encouraged him to look at his bowel flora because of the profound impact gut bacteria have on mood.

There is abundant evidence of a gut–brain connection that is not solely mediated by the immune system. This means that although it is easy to understand that gut inflammation would cause it to leak and contribute to widespread ravages affecting the brain and behaviour, research has also highlighted that even when the gut is intact, there are clear reciprocal (neurological) interactions between gut bacteria and mental state. Stress can damage our healthy bacterial colonies, while encouraging the proliferation of lactobacillus and bifidus bacteria will positively impact on mood and behaviour.

We agreed to use a strong probiotic supplement twice daily and Stuart started to add fermented vegetables to his diet. I also worked with him to regularly implant acidophilus directly into his colon via a small catheter. This, combined with the help of a counsellor recommended by his GP, meant that six months later he was finally free from his addiction and much calmer, having also reduced his coffee intake.

SOPHIE'S STORY
POOR DIET AND IRREGULAR HOURS

Sophie is an actress. She has gained a reputation for playing the older sister in period dramas. She is known for her complexion and her figure which she accentuates beautifully with a slightly provocative demeanour. She oozes understated sex appeal and this has ensured she gets regular parts providing she keeps a tight hold on her weight and physical appearance. Acting is not a glamorous job. You have to be on set at all hours of the day or night and be prepared to seemingly wait patiently to make your brief, but essential, appearance. Food is provided by catering companies that are less concerned about health than transportability. Boredom can set in and wear down good intentions, while lack of routine can disrupt the body clock and create stress. As a result, Sophie was either on a starvation diet or sugar bingeing.

Since her fortieth birthday the latter had become a more regular feature. When I met her she had gained eight pounds and her self-esteem was low. A number of my clients come to see me claiming to want to detox but what they really mean to say is, "I want to lose weight quickly, look 10 years younger and feel confident again." In many ways those are realistic expectations from a healthier diet and a more functional lifestyle (as outlined in this book) but, 'quick' is a relative concept. If it took 15 years to gradually put on 10kg, one year is a very short time to lose it and to think otherwise would be a mistake, because detoxing can quickly start to look like a cycle of binge/starvation.

Detox is less about weight loss than working with our physiology to improve how we feel, which in turn drives our inner equilibrium and behaviour. Unless we take ownership of our body in its entirety we cannot begin to work with it in a functional and therapeutic way. This is what I explained to Sophie before telling her that she had to eat more calories in the form of fat. Her sugar-bingeing habit may have provided her with the stated calories for her metabolism but instead of training her body to burn fat it was training it to lay fat. Especially because she had also trained it to expect periods of starvation for which storage came useful. In fact this mechanism had successfully ensured the survival of her ancestors through famines and long winters. This made sense to her and Sophie agreed to look at fat differently.

For breakfast and lunch I recommended that she use a whey protein shake to which she added ground flax, a large tablespoon of coconut oil, lecithin and a multi green/probiotic powdered blend. For taste I told her to experiment with various berries (available frozen or freeze-dried), vanilla essence, lucuma powder and cacao powder. I also encouraged her to use gelatine to make 'set smoothies'. This would add interest and variety as well as provide skin-firming benefits from the collagen in gelatine. In this way she would not have depend on caterers as much and could still enjoy a meal in the evening which she frequently would have at a restaurant.

I also discussed strategies with Sophie to help her fill the waiting time productively. In particular, she had to learn basic movements that could be done with minimum space to ensure that she kept moving. I told her about the importance of sleep in regulating appetite and sugar cravings and insisted that she avoid strictly all junk food and sugar. Instead she could nibble on nuts, vegetable sticks and cherry tomatoes. Fruits were permitted if they were fresh and limited to three pieces per day. Whenever Sophie had a very relaxing pampering day available, I told her that was the time to practise juice fasting and only drink vegetable juices that day. I asked her to report back two months later, however, I heard nothing until almost a year later. By then she had embraced detox, raw food and healthy eating so much that she wanted to train in nutrition and was looking for a course in raw-food preparation.

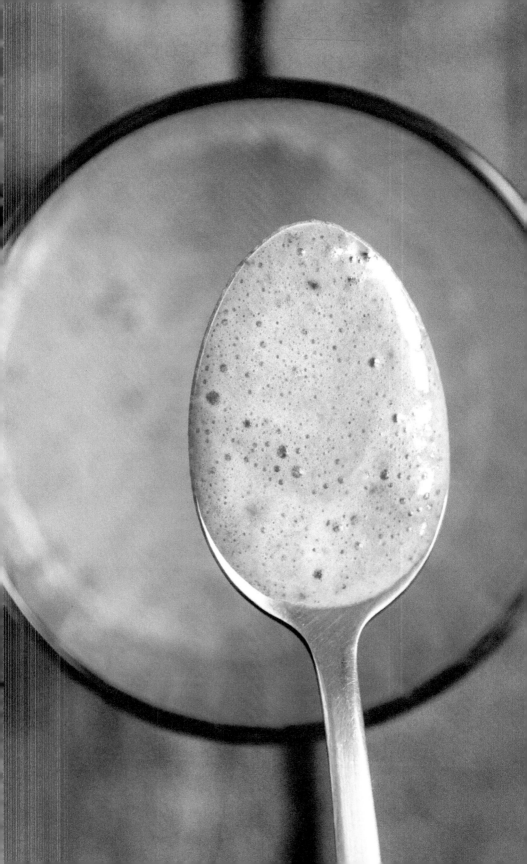

PART SIX:
RECIPES

"It should be a simple matter to eat in such a way that the greatest possible health of body and spirit results."

DR RALPH BIRCHER,
Bircher-Benner Clinic

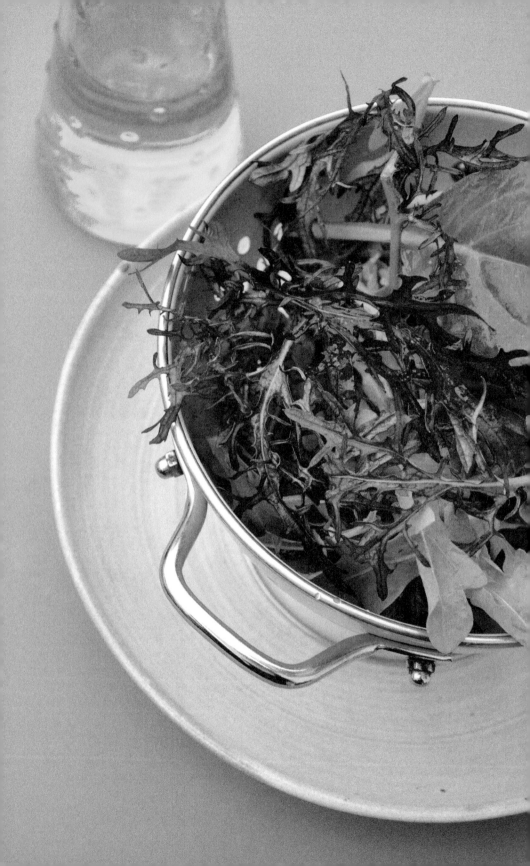

RECIPES

DETOX RECIPES

JUICING

Juicing is one of the best ways to extract and concentrate nutrients and antioxidants from fruits and vegetables. Unlike smoothies, juices contain very little fibre, require minimal digestion and are easily and quickly absorbed, thus delivering nourishment straight to the cells.

There are two basic ways to extract juices from fruits and vegetable. The more common, quicker and cheaper method uses centrifugal speed, the other uses a slow mechanical process – these are sometimes called masticating juicers. Both systems have advantages but masticating-juicer technology has progressed and prices have dropped in the last couple of years, making this type of juicer my preferred choice. They are slower than centrifugal juicers but for personal and family consumption they are fast enough and generally quicker to clean. They can also produce juice from leafy vegetables like spinach and softer fruits like papaya or berries without wasting most of it. The pulp that comes out is much drier than with conventional centrifugal juicers, making them more economical in the long run. They also produce a juice that oxidises less quickly and which can be kept in a sealed (glass) container for up to 12 hours in the fridge. Adding lemon juice also helps with preventing oxidisation.

Most fruits and vegetables do not need to be peeled before juicing. However citrus skin can be toxic in large quantities. Make sure to scrub the skin of non-organic produce.

If you are using a centrifugal juicer, try pushing the soft, leafy ingredients in small amounts together with harder ingredients like apples or carrots.

If you are using a masticating juicer, this is not necessary and you can expand your repertoire to include juices made from spinach, Swiss chard, dandelion leaves, beet tops, etc

As with smoothies, fewer ingredients make fresh juices more tasty. Lemon juice is a great ingredient for adjusting the taste of bland juices such as carrots and ginger will liven up any juice. Fruit juices are helpful for improving taste, but make sure not to overdo the fruits as they are very high in sugar.

The following are ideas to get you started. By using organic seasonal fruit and vegetables means that you will get the most from your juicing effort and this may mean that you will have to experiment!

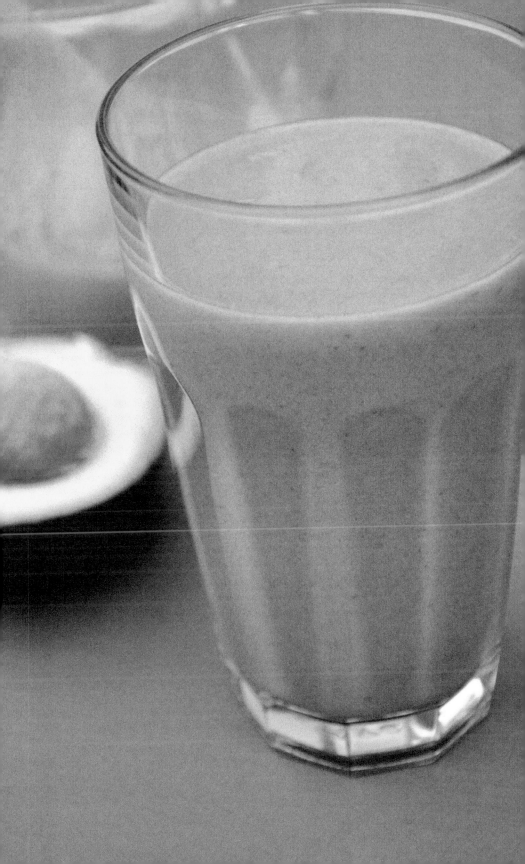

Some juice ideas to get you started:
Liver (detox) juice #1: Beetroot, carrot, grapefruit
Liver (balancing) juice #2: Broccoli stalk, apple, lime, ginger root
Liver (nourishing) juice #3: Carrot, coriander, orange, turmeric or ginger root

Kidney (balancing) juice #1: Celery, apple, lemon, ginger
Kidney (detox/diuretic) juice #2: Fennel, parsley, celery, grapefruit
Kidney (nourishing) juice #3: Cucumber, lime, mint

Cleansing juice #1: Beetroot, orange, spinach
Cleansing juice #2: Kiwi, cucumber, kale
Cleansing juice #3: Tomato, sweet pepper, carrot, celery

MAKING HEALTHFUL AND TASTY SMOOTHIES

Smoothies are quick and easy to make. They are transportable, and depending on ingredients, can be consumed as a meal replacement. If you are going to make smoothies regularly, I recommend that you invest in a smoothie maker or a strong blender. A basic food processor with a liquidiser may not be sturdy enough for chopping vegetables.

Specialised appliances also double up as a grinder for nuts and seeds. They can be used to chop herbs, blend batter, hummus and guacamole, and to mix ingredients for fruit, nut and protein bars/snacks.

Green smoothies combine green leafy vegetables, with other superfoods like spirulina, whey and pollen. Some green vegetables such as kale* or broccoli and powdered greens can be quite potent in flavour, but as long as your smoothie has a strong fruity element it will override all these 'green' flavours. The consistency of a smoothie is important. Enhance it by adding a creamy element like nut butter, avocado or coconut oil. Fat improves consistency and increases the absorption of the precious chlorophyll and antioxidants in greens. Together with protein, fat also helps curb hunger and cravings.

A green smoothie is an ideal way to deliver easily digested nutrition and increase fibre in the diet while reducing cravings. Unfortunately smoothies oxidise quickly. If you do not intend to drink yours straightaway, add ½ tsp of ascorbic acid (powdered vitamin C) to preserve the delicate nutrients. Invest in a cooling container and make sure that you consume your smoothie within four hours of blending.

Follow the basic guidelines (FGF+F) to build your own green smoothie recipe. In a blender combine:

- **F** – ⅓ fruit element such as cucumber, tomato, sweet pepper, citrus, berries, pineapple, mango, banana, peach, papaya, pear, etc
- **G** – ⅓ green and leafy element. Vary between kale (best lightly steamed for a couple of minutes to eliminate the anti-nutrients that are present in raw kale which interfere with thyroid function), spinach, lamb's lettuce, parsley, coriander, lettuce of any kind, mint, sorrel, rocket, chard, beet tops, dandelion leaves, young stinging nettle leaves, etc Leafy vegetables are especially rich in antioxidants because they have to photosynthesise without getting damaged by the sun's radiation. They also contain chemicals designed to protect them from fungi, bacteria and pests. This is in contrast to the fruit plants dependent on micro-organisms or being eaten (by birds for instance) for dissemination. Those phytochemicals (otherwise known as anti-nutrients) can stop the absorption of essential minerals and are potentially toxic; in humans they are usually dealt with by our gut flora, providing it is appropriate and matches requirements. It is important not to overdo green leaves (especially if you are not used to it and have not yet built the appropriate flora) and it is essential to rotate them to avoid the accumulation of a particular anti-nutrient.
- **F** – ⅓ fatty element and superfoods combined. The fatty element can be a couple of tablespoons of avocado, almond butter, hemp seed oil, coconut oil, cashew nuts, etc The superfood element can be a tsp of spirulina, ground turmeric, bee pollen or lecithin, and/or a tablespoon of whey protein or ground flax.
- **+F** – To improve the taste you can also use specific flavouring elements such as vanilla essence, cacao or freeze dried berry powder (blueberry, strawberry, acai berry, raspberry, etc).

I recommend that you don't use too many ingredients – it can quickly become an indistinct and muddy concoction. To guarantee your diet contains regular health-enhancing superfoods, rotate ingredients and take pleasure in your smoothie.

POTASSIUM BROTH

Potassium broth is a rich source of minerals. Minerals control water balance, neurological and muscular function as well as aiding detox. Potassium must be plentiful to balance out sodium (salt). Additional potassium is particularly useful during a detox to help the kidneys buffer the acids released by the process of detoxification and is found in fresh fruit and vegetables.

Make the broth by simmering vegetables together for 1–3 hours. Use dark green leafy kale, spinach, beet tops, radish tops, watercress (you can use some of the vegetable mush that comes out of your juicer) with herbs, garlic and spices of your choice. Season with kelp powder, miso or Atlantic/Himalayan salt and strain it through a fine sieve. Drink the warm liquid throughout the day as part of a juice fast and whenever a warm savoury tea is called for.

To increase potassium content you can add potato peelings to your mix. Traditional potassium broth was made with potato peelings alone and a little seasoning but this is far from palatable!!

FERMENTED FOODS

The type of fermentation that interests us in terms of probiotic organisms is called lacto-fermentation and is characterised by the type of friendly bacteria broadly referred to as lactobacillus. Fermentation is their way of mobilising energy from various sugars in the absence of oxygen. The by-product of their fermentation is lactic acid which is what gives fermented products their acidic flavour and also ensures that other (putrefactive) bacteria are not able to survive. Indeed lacto-fermentation is one of the safest ways to preserve food and it effectively sustained our forefathers and mothers before fridges were invented.

FERMENTING VEGETABLES

Lactobacillus are abundant in the soil and found on the skin of vegetables that are close to the ground such as cabbages and carrots. They are sensitive to pesticides, herbicides and chlorine (from tap water). It is therefore essential to choose organic for all your fermented vegetable recipes.

Fermenting vegetables is not complicated. It is more of an art than a science and you can develop your own technique and method.

There are three fundamental steps:

1. **The pre-fermentation stage:** lasts 2–3 days. It is the complicated phase when the various colonies are getting established. The vegetables are beginning to soften and decompose. It is possible to influence bacteria types by adding a commercial probiotic to the mix at this stage.
2. **The acidifying stage:** this is when the lactic acid bacteria colonies start to dominate and take over their acid-sensitive neighbours. After 2–3 weeks only the lactic acid bacteria remain and after 3–5 weeks the lacto-fermenting bacteria stop multiplying and this phase is completed. During

that time vitamins and co-nutrients are also created as part of the process, contributing further to the nutritional quality of fermented vegetables.

3. **The stocking stage,** which can take place when the pH has reached a value inferior to 4.1 and can last up to a year.

There are three specific controlling factors that will ensure the successful fermentation of vegetables:

1. **Temperature:** ideally it should be around 20°C in the first stage but should be a few degrees lower during the acidifying phase and cool or cold for the stocking phase.
2. **Oxygen:** must be completely eliminated by fully immersing the vegetables. If not, yeast will be able to develop.
3. **Salt concentration:** should be between 0.5% and 2% of the vegetable weight. Salt is not essential; however, it helps to acidify the environment from the start and it prevents the decomposition of the protein in the vegetables which keeps them more crunchy.

Sauerkraut

Cabbage is traditionally fermented to make sauerkraut. It needs to be organic unwashed (outer leaves removed), finely sliced and the core discarded.

- Weigh the cabbage and use 10% of that weight in salt.
- Prepare the jars (mason jars or fermenting crock or rubber sealed jars are all suitable) by sterilising them in a dishwasher or oven.
- With clean hands massage the salt and cabbage together. You can also add coriander seeds, cumin, fresh garlic cloves, etc to your mix.
- Pack your jars very carefully, making sure that the cabbage shreds are pushed down with your fist at every layer and that all the air is pushed out.
- Stop packing 2.5cm (1 inch) below the top and close your jar.
- Leave it on a plate and let phase one develop.
- After a few hours the cabbage will emit its water, covering all the layers, and the process will have started. Don't be tempted to open the jar even if it overflows.
- After a week you can transfer the jar to a cooler place like a cellar and let it develop for 5–6 weeks. The colder the ambient temperature, the slower the process is. The sauerkraut should be ready to consume after 6 weeks and should have a pleasant smell. If this is not the case something went wrong and you will not want to eat it!

This procedure can be followed with any vegetables: beetroot, turnip, swede, carrot, celery, etc. Whole baby vegetables (not cherry tomatoes) and garlic cloves can be fermented but will have to be covered in non-chlorinated water before fermenting. Add the juice of a lemon and the required amount of salt (10% of the vegetable weight). You can also include a cinnamon stick, whole cloves, juniper berries, herbs and spices before closing the jar. After a week, you can open it to remove the scum from the top. Reseal to complete the process.

FERMENTING MILK AND MAKING YOGHURT

- Yoghurt and similar cultured milk (kefir, buttermilk etc) can be made from dairy, soya or nut milk. They require the appropriate starter culture to achieve the desired result and you will need to buy this from a specialised supplier. Different cultures produce different setting qualities and some, like kefir, don't set at all. It is possible to use a commercial yoghurt for the starter but by the time you buy it the viability of the bacteria is often much reduced and unlikely to produce a good result.
- All yoghurts are made in the same way but nut yoghurt (coconut in particular) will remain runny unless you use a gelling agent like gelatine or agar-agar seaweed. Dissolve in boiling water and add to the warmed-up milk, stirring thoroughly.

The secret to making yoghurt is to heat the milk to the correct temperature (50°C) and to maintain it at a warm temperature for 8 hours after that for the bacteria to thrive. The bacteria will be killed if you go much over 55°C and will not get established unless the milk is warm. Yoghurt makers are useful for this although with a thermometer, a pan and a wide-mouth thermo-flask it is possible to achieve good results.

FERMENTING GRAINS

Grains are easily fermented and this is the process involved in making sourdough. Unlike vegetables, the fermenting organisms are collected from the surroundings more than from the grains themselves.

Rejuvelac

This is made by letting 1 cup of organic wheat beads sprout for 24–36hours before blending with 3 cups of water and immersing in 1½ of filtered water. Leave the jar uncovered to ferment in a clean, warm place. Allow fermentation for 2-5 days before filtering and transferring to the fridge in a sealed container. Rejuvelac can be used as a starter for making nut yoghurt, flavouring in pancake batter or drunk as a probiotic drink. It can be improved by seeding it with a commercial probiotic.

FERMENTING NUTS AND SEEDS
- Nuts and seeds are fermented with rejuvelac as a starter and make seed or nut 'cheeses'.
- Cashew nuts and sunflower seeds are the common ones used to make those vegan 'cheeses'.

CASHEW NUT CHEESE

INGREDIENTS
2 cups cashew nuts
½ cup rejuvelac
Dash of sea salt
Dried herbs/cracked pepper to coat

METHOD
1. Cover the cashews with water and soak overnight. Drain.
2. Place the cashews in a food processor and blend with the rejuvelac until a smooth paste forms.
3. Season with sea salt to taste.
4. Line a strainer with 2 layers of cheesecloth.
5. Spoon the mixture into the cloth. Set in a warm place and leave for 24 to 36 hours over a large bowl
6. Form the cheese into rounds or logs and coat the outside with herbs or cracked pepper.
7. Put in refrigerator to set.
8. This 'cheese' will keep in the refrigerator for about a week.

SUNFLOWER CREAM CHEESE

INGREDIENTS
1 cup unhulled sunflower seeds
½ cup rejuvelac
1 tbsp tahini (sesame butter)
Herb, seaweeds and garlic mix of your choice
½ tsp miso

METHOD
1. Soak the seeds overnight in chlorine-free or filtered water. Drain and rinse in filtered water.
2. Place in a food processor and blend with the rejuvelac, tahini and herb mixture until a smooth paste forms
3. Season with miso (or sea salt)
4. Leave in a warm place to ferment for 6–8 hours. Taste to check timing.
5. Spoon the mixture into a sealed container and refrigerate.

BASIC BREADS, MUFFINS AND WRAP RECIPES

By using an alternative ingredient, they are designed to be high in health-enhancing nutrients, fibre and protein and low in sugar and carbohydrates. This makes them nourishing and satisfying without a negative impact on blood sugar.

TWO-INGREDIENT BANANA PANCAKES
(Makes 2–3 pancakes, depending on pan size)

You've guessed it, these are made with banana and eggs. However some optional extras can be added. A favourite of mine, they make a quick snack when in a hurry or when you only have two ingredients left in your fridge!

INGREDIENTS
1 medium ripe banana
2 medium eggs
¼ tsp baking powder, for added lightness
50ml oat milk (optional) for thinner/lighter pancakes
¼ cup (30g) ground almonds, for added consistency and taste

METHOD
1. Mash the banana with a fork and mix with the eggs, or use a blender and whisk all the ingredients together into a thinner batter.
2. Preheat a skillet or small (ceramic) pan and brush with (coconut) butter to prevent sticking.
3. Drop the batter into the pan (2–3 tablespoons depending on consistency)
4. Wait until the pancake is set before turning over with a thin spatula.
5. Cook on the other side for a further minute or so.
6. Repeat with remaining batter.

ARROWROOT GLUTEN-FREE WRAP
(Makes 6–8 wraps, depending on pan size)

The arrowroot flour makes these pliable. They can be bent, rolled and folded without tearing. They work well with a sweet filling like stewed apples and cinnamon and are excellent for savoury wraps like chicken, shrimp or tuna salad. Once made, they can can be frozen, or kept refrigerated for up to 4 days.

INGREDIENTS

⅓ cup (50g) arrowroot powder (available from health stores and some supermarkets)
4 eggs
200ml water or almond milk
Pinch of salt
Butter, to brush pan

METHOD

1. In a blender or bowl whisk all the ingredients (except the butter) together into a watery batter

2. Brush a frying pan (a small ceramic frying pan is ideal because it is perfectly non-stick and non-toxic) with butter and preheat for 2 minutes over a medium heat.

3. Pour a small ladleful of the batter into the hot pan and spread it by tilting the pan. It should start to cook as soon as you do that. When the batter is solid flip the wrap with a spatula and cook on the other side for 30 seconds.

4. Slide onto a warmed plate and repeat with the remaining batter.

OAT BRAN AND PUMPKIN MUFFINS
(Makes 6 muffins)

Muffins are portable and make a great snack when on the move. These contain oat bran (a good source of fibre) which makes them denser and more like traditional muffins. They are also rich in healthful spices and can be made sweeter by adding raisins or more savoury by adding olives and replacing the spices with mixed herbs.

INGREDIENTS
½ cup (50g) ground almonds
½ cup (60g) oat bran
Mixed spice: ½ tsp cinnamon, ¼ tsp ginger, ¼ tsp cloves, ¼ tsp nutmeg, ¼ tsp turmeric (adjusted to your taste or use 2 tsp allspice)
½ tsp salt
1 tsp baking powder
1 cup (225g) mashed pumpkin, tinned pumpkin or winter squash
3 medium eggs
2 tbsp (30g) melted (coconut) oil/butter
½ cup (50g) chopped walnuts (optional)
⅓ cup (60g) dates or raisins (optional)
Grated coconut

METHOD
1. Preheat the oven to 320°F/160°C /fan oven 140°C/gas mark 3
2. In a food processor (I use the blade accessory) mix the dry ingredients first – the ground almonds, oat bran, spices, salt and baking powder.
3. Add the wet ingredients – the mashed pumpkin or squash, eggs and melted coconut oil/ butter) and continue to mix thoroughly.
4. If using, fold in by hand the walnuts and dates or raisins.
5. Spoon the batter into a lined (or silicone) 6-hole muffin tin; only three quarters full to allow for them to rise
6. Top with the grated coconut
7. Bake for 35 minutes or until cooked through. Check by piercing one with a knife, if it comes out clean, they are ready.
8. Take out of the tin when warm and allow to cool completely before serving (if you can wait that long!)

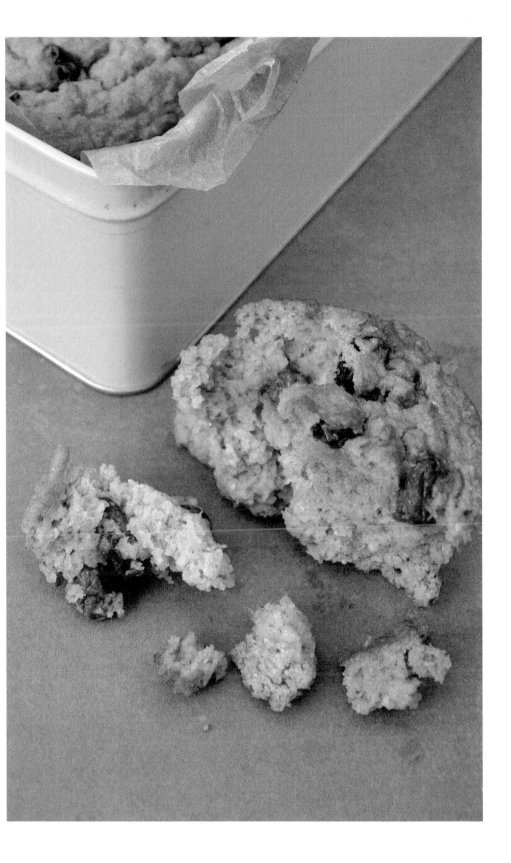

CARB-FREE COCONUT FLOUR BREAD
A satisfying and moist alternative to bread (Serves 6–8)

INGREDIENTS

½ cup (60g) coconut flour
½ tsp salt
1 tsp thyme (optional)
1 tsp baking soda
4 medium eggs
3 tbsp. (45g) melted (coconut) butter
2 tsp apple cider vinegar
4 medium carrots (or 2 large courgettes), grated*
½ cup of broken walnuts, plus a few walnut halves to decorate

*If you would like to make more of a cake use grated apples instead of the vegetables and cinnamon instead of thyme.

METHOD

1. Preheat the oven to 320°F/160°C /fan oven 140°C/gas mark 3
2. In a mixing bowl, mix the dry ingredients – the coconut flour, salt, thyme and baking soda.
3. In a blender, mix the eggs, melted (coconut) butter and apple cider vinegar.
4. Add the dry ingredients to the blender and mix to combine into a thick batter.
5. Transfer the batter into a bowl and fold in by hand the grated vegetables and walnuts.
6. Pour into a greased loaf tin that has been lined with parchment paper (or a silicone bread mould) and decorate with walnut halves or grated coconut.
7. Bake for 40 minutes or until cooked through. Check by piercing one with a knife, if it comes out clean, they are ready.
8. Take out of the tin while warm and allow to cool completely before serving.

FLOURLESS BANANA AND PROTEIN LOAF
(Makes I loaf)

This banana loaf is moist and the perfect accompaniment to an afternoon tea. It can be enjoyed by everyone yet, unlike cakes and biscuits, will not cause excessively high blood sugar. Add stevia if you would like to make it sweeter.

INGREDIENTS

1½ cups (150g) ground almonds or hazelnuts
½ cup (50g) whole chia seeds
⅔ cup (60g) whey protein isolate
1 tsp baking soda
½ tsp sea salt
½ tsp cinnamon or allspice
2 large eggs
3 medium and very ripe mashed bananas
200ml almond milk or water
1 tbsp vanilla extract

METHOD

1. Preheat oven to 320°F/160°C /(fan oven 140°C)/gas mark 3
2. In a mixing bowl mix all the dry ingredients – ground almonds, chia, whey, baking soda, salt and spices.
3. Separate the egg whites from yolks and beat until stiff and fluffy. Reserve.
4. In a food processor (I used the blade accessory) or a blender, mix the egg yolks, banana, almond milk or water and vanilla.
5. Add the dry ingredients and continue to mix thoroughly to the consistency of a thick batter.
6. Transfer into a bowl and fold in the egg whites
7. Pour into a greased loaf tin that has been lined with parchment paper (or a silicone bread mould)
8. Bake for 40–50 minutes or until cooked through. Check by piercing with a knife, if it comes out clean, it's ready.
9. Take out of the tin while warm and allow to cool completely before serving

ANTI-INFLAMMATORY AND CARDIOVASCULAR HEALTH RECIPES

TURMERIC AND GINGER

Have been shown to help turn off NF-kB, a protein that regulates the immune system and triggers the process of inflammation. Ginger has also been shown to reduce intestinal inflammation.

OILY FISH

Salmon, mackerel, sardines, trout and herring are high in long-chain omega-3 fatty acids, which play an important role in heart disease prevention and help control inflammation.

GARLIC AND ONIONS

Garlic in particular has been shown to shut off pathways leading to inflammation in a similar way to non-steroid pain medications. Onions and garlic both contain anti-inflammatory antioxidants like quercetin and allicin, which break down into sulfenic acid, a powerful free-radical scavenger. However, for some people this can be a difficult conversion leading to intolerances and abdominal bloating.

BEETROOT AND CHARD

Contain specific pigments called betalains which have been shown to reduce inflammation, as well as protect against cancer and heart disease.

BERRIES

Are very rich in anthocyanins, powerful antioxidants that give them their rich colour and have been shown to reduce inflammation and support cardiovascular health. Studies have shown, for example, that red raspberry extract helped prevent animals from developing arthritis; that blueberries can help protect against intestinal inflammation and ulcerative colitis; and that women who eat more strawberries have lower levels of C-reactive protein (inflammation marker) in their blood. Berries will enhance many sweet and savoury recipes from yoghurt and smoothies to salads and venison dishes.

ONION MARMALADE
(Makes 4 x 250ml jars)

INGREDIENTS

3 tbsp butter
1kg red or white onions, finely sliced
2 tbsp molasses, honey or brown sugar (optional)
150ml red wine vinegar
125ml port (or red wine)
2 tbsp arrowroot
Sea salt and ground black pepper

METHOD

1. Heat the butter in a large heavy-based pan.
2. Add the onions and cook gently, stirring regularly, until very soft and slightly caramelising– approximately 30 minutes.
3. Add the molasses, vinegar and port and simmer to reduce for a further 45 minutes
4. Meanwhile, sterilise the jars by putting them on a baking tray and into a cold oven. Heat to 284°F/140°C/fan oven 120°C/gas mark 1 for 15 minutes.
5. Mix the arrowroot with a little of the hot liquid from the pot before stirring it back in and cooking for a further 10 minutes while stirring continuously. Season to taste.
6. Pour the hot onion mixture into the hot jars straight from the oven. Fill them right to the top and use a skewer to poke out any air holes. Then screw on the lids and turn upside down for 15 minutes to sterilise the lids.
7. Let the jars cool down and store in a dry place. Consume within 3 months. Once you have open a jar it must be kept refrigerated and eaten within 2 weeks.

BEETROOT WEDGES AND SPICY MAYO DIP
(Serves 2)

INGREDIENTS

For the wedges:
4 large beetroot
2 tbsp. (30g) coconut oil (it may need warming up slightly to liquify it)
½ tsp of turmeric
I clove crushed garlic
Salt and pepper to season

For the spicy mayo dip:
200ml plain bio (goat's) yoghurt
I garlic clove
½ tsp ground ginger OR 2.5cm or I inch fresh peeled ginger
½ tsp ground turmeric
I raw egg yolk or I tsp liquid lecithin
Salt and pepper, to taste
Chopped fresh parsley, to garnish

METHOD

1. Preheat the oven to 356°F/180°C /fan oven 160°C/gas mark 4.
2. Peel the beetroot and cut into equal-sized wedges.
3. Place the wedges in a bowl and
4. pour over the oil, turmeric and seasoning.
5. Toss well so that they are evenly coated.
6. Spread on a large baking tray and bake in oven for 35–45 minutes, or until the wedges are soft in the middle and crispy on the outside.
7. Combine the mayo ingredients in a blender
8. Serve the wedges straight from the oven with the mayo dip and garnished with chopped parsley. Combines perfectly with baked salmon

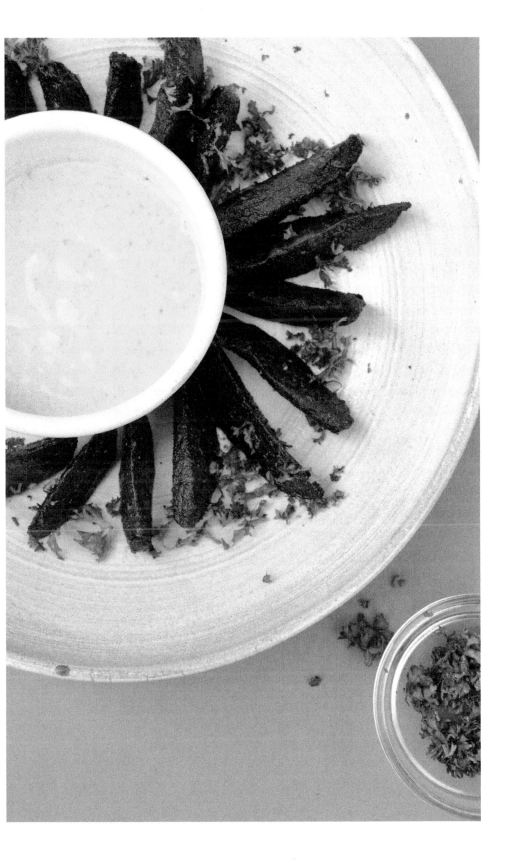

PROSTATE HEALTH RECIPES

TOMATOES
Rich in the antioxidant lycopene, which has been shown to lower the risk of developing prostate cancer. According to the National Cancer Institute it reduces symptoms associated with benign prostatic hypertrophy (BPH). Lycopene has also been shown to lower the blood levels of the prostate-specific antigen (PSA) connected with prostatic inflammation and BPH.

PUMPKIN SEEDS AND AVOCADO
Are rich in the fatty acid beta-sitosterol, a plant sterol. According to the *Cochrane Database of Systematic Reviews,* beta-sitosterol can help reduce symptoms associated with BPH. Men taking beta-sitosterol supplements have better urinary flow and less residual urine volume.

SAW PALMETTO
Contains high levels of different kinds of sitosterols which counteract prostate enlargement. Saw palmetto has been shown to block the enzyme that converts testosterone to prolactin and causes prostate enlargement in older men, thus preserving healthy testosterone levels. Saw palmetto is thought to strengthen the male reproductive organs and boost sexual appetite. Do not combine with anti-androgenic medications.

ARGAN OIL
One of the richest sources of vitamin E. Argan oil has been shown to decrease the proliferation rate of prostate cancer cells. A 2006 study in *Cancer Investigation* reported that fatty acid components of argan oil slowed the growth of several types of prostate cancer cells. Exposure to those components was also able to reverse the cancerous effect of carcinogens on prostate cells.

TOMATO SAUCE
(Makes sauce for 2)

INGREDIENTS

1 carrot
1 red pepper
1 deseeded jalapeño
pepper, add a little
more if you like it spicy
3 large tomatoes
1 celery stalk
Large handful of fresh
basil leaves
1 tbsp dried mixed
herbs (oregano,
rosemary, thyme)
1 tbsp apple cider
vinegar (or a juiced
lime)
1 tbsp argan oil
Salt and pepper to taste

METHOD

1. Peel the carrot and deseed the peppers before cutting all the vegetables into chunks.
2. Place the vegetables and herbs in a saucepan, cover with lid and simmer for about 20 minutes or until all vegetables are soft.
3. Using a hand-held blender, blend until smooth.
4. Add the apple cider vinegar (it will help keep the colour bright) and argan oil. Season to taste.
5. Simmer gently for a further 20 minutes to reduce.
6. Serve with oven-baked salmon fillets.

GUACAMOLE (AVOCADO DIP) WITH SAW PALMETTO & ARGAN OIL
(Makes 1 bowl or 2 servings)

INGREDIENTS

4 very ripe avocados
2 tsp powdered saw
palmetto berries*
8 cherry tomatoes
Handful of fresh
coriander
2 tbsp argan oil
½ tsp ground turmeric
3 limes
Salt to season

METHOD

1. Scoop the avocados and place in a blender with all the remaining ingredients.
2. Serve with grilled or raw vegetable sticks (broccoli, cauliflower, sweet potatoes, fennel, carrots, peppers, mushrooms, asparagus, courgettes (zucchini), etc)

*Available to order from Indigo Herbs http://www.indigo-herbs.co.uk/

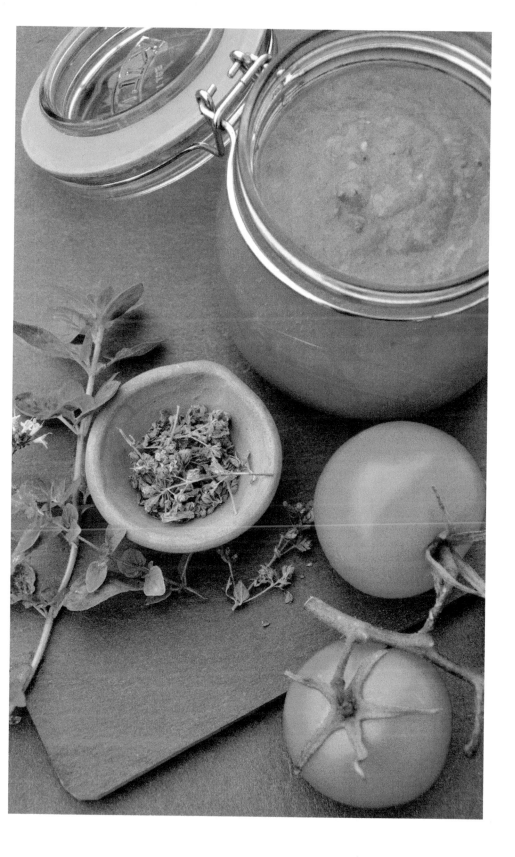

RECIPES FOR STRONG BONES, NAILS AND HAIR

GELATINE

Contains collagen and hyaluronic acid, two important constituents of connective tissues, bones and ligaments. They contribute to skin elasticity and hair and nail growth. Collagen supplementation has been shown to reduce wrinkles and improve bone and joint health.

SILICA

Silica is not a common trace mineral. Millet and cucumber are the best sources. It can be converted to calcium by the body and contribute to connective tissue growth and maintenance. It has been shown to help improve hair and nail health.

KELP

Kelp is a great thyroid support and a rich source of iodine. One of the first symptoms of low thyroid function is hair loss, especially the outer third of the eyebrows.

IRON

Iron deficiency and anaemia also cause hair loss and often go hand in hand with low thyroid function. Iron supplementation is not recommended as it causes constipation and can lead to iron toxicity. If possible aim to increase iron levels naturally by eating organic liver instead, or drinking iron-rich mineral water (Spatone is available from health shops).

BONE BROTH

Bone broth or consomme is a cheap and effective way to extract collagen and minerals from animal bones. The quality and proportions of those precious elements makes them especially well absorbed and ensures delivery to our own connective tissues and bones. This is the recipe I recommend to anyone with joint or bone problems and to improve skin elasticity and prevent sagging. Bone broth is also a great source of the amino acids glycine, proline and glutamine and is very healing to the gut lining. This is consistent with the traditional use of chicken soup as an immune system booster and (digestive) cure all.

You can make bone broth using whole organic chicken, whole fish or fish bones (including the fish head), pork or beef bones. Each will render a different flavour. I suggest starting with chicken because it has the mildest flavour.

If you are using chicken, simply place the entire raw chicken into a large pot and cover with water. Add 60ml of apple cider vinegar to help leach the minerals from the bones. Alternatively, you can use a leftover carcass from a roasted chicken. Don't be afraid to add the feet and the head, as they're great sources of collagen. Pig's feet are one of the richest sources of collagen.

Bring it all to a boil. At this stage the liquid is typically skimmed. This is, however, not necessary; the scum that rises to the top of the stock pot — although off-putting — is a rich source of amino acids. Once it is boiling, turn down the heat and let it simmer for 4–24 hours. The longer the better, and an electric slowcooker is an excellent way to safely achieve this. Ideally you want the bones to become soft.

You can also add vegetables of your choice and a small tsp of powdered kelp, salt, pepper, spices and herbs into the pot.

Once your broth is cooked you can scoop the liquid with a ladle and serve it as it is. However, in order to keep it or freeze it you will have to strain it through a fine-mesh colander and separate the liquid. Do this over a large bowl and express all the liquid by compressing the solids through the colander and leaving it to drip for 15 minutes. Once you have collected the consommé you can use it as a stock for cooking soup or consume it as a salty and tasty tea.

MILLET TABOULI
(Serves 2–3)

INGREDIENTS

1 cup (200g) millet
1 tbsp coconut oil
100ml water, stock or bone broth
1 large cucumber
1 small red onion
3 tomatoes
Bunch of fresh mint
5 tbsp olive oil
15-30 olives – chopped
Juice of 1 lemon
Salt and pepper, to taste

METHOD

1. Soak the millet for 2 hours to release anti-nutrients and improve silica absorption.
2. Rinse, place in a pan with the oil and toast for 2 minutes.
3. Add the water or stock, cover and cook over a low heat for 20 minutes or until soft.
4. Dice the cucumber, onion and tomatoes and finely chop the mint leaves (retain a few sprigs for garnish).
5. Combine the cooked millet with the vegetables and all the remaining ingredients
6. Toss together well and serve garnished with the mint sprigs.

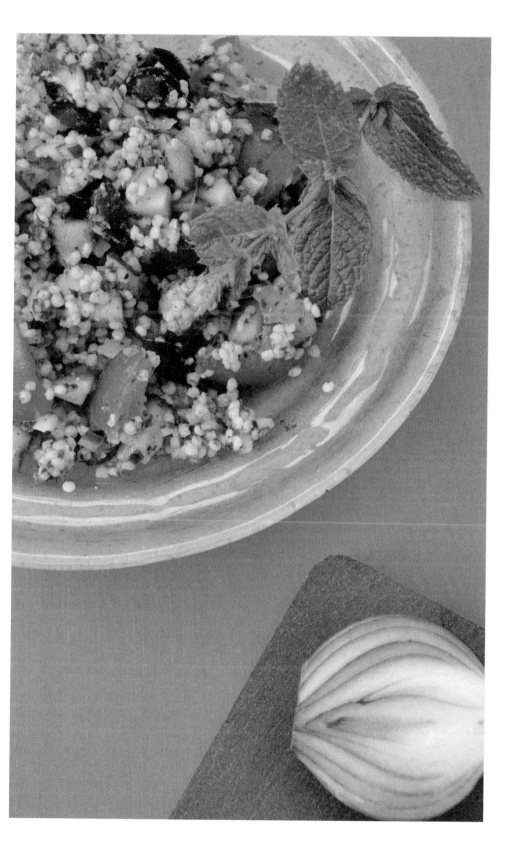

EASY MENOPAUSE RECIPES

KUDZU
Contains a number of isoflavone compounds (phytoestrogen) that can alleviate menopausal symptoms including hot flushes and night sweats. A study published in the July 2007 issue of the *Journal of the Medical Association of Thailand* showed that kudzu helps alleviate hot flushes and night sweats. Research findings published in the July 2003 of *Menopause* also found that kudzu may improve cognitive function in women who have been through the menopause.

ALFALFA
A natural source of progesterone and phytoestrogen. It is used traditionally used to promote better hormonal balance during menopause and has been shown to increase blood progesterone levels. Alfalfa sprouts are a delicious addition to salads.

FLAX SEEDS
The richest source of lignans, an isoflavone which appears to reduce blood sugar levels and menopausal symptoms like hot flushes and mood swings.

CRUCIFEROUS VEGETABLES
Cruciferous vegetables (broccoli, turnips, Brussels sprouts, cabbage, pak choi, Chinese cabbage, rocket, collard greens, horseradish, kale, kohlrabi, radishes, mustard greens, rutabaga, wasabi, daikon and watercress) are rich sources of sulphur-containing compounds known as glucosinolates which have been shown to reduce oestrogen toxicity and protect against (hormone-dependent) cancers.

SAGE
A traditional herb used in the treatment of menopause which has been clinically proven to alleviate excessive sweating.

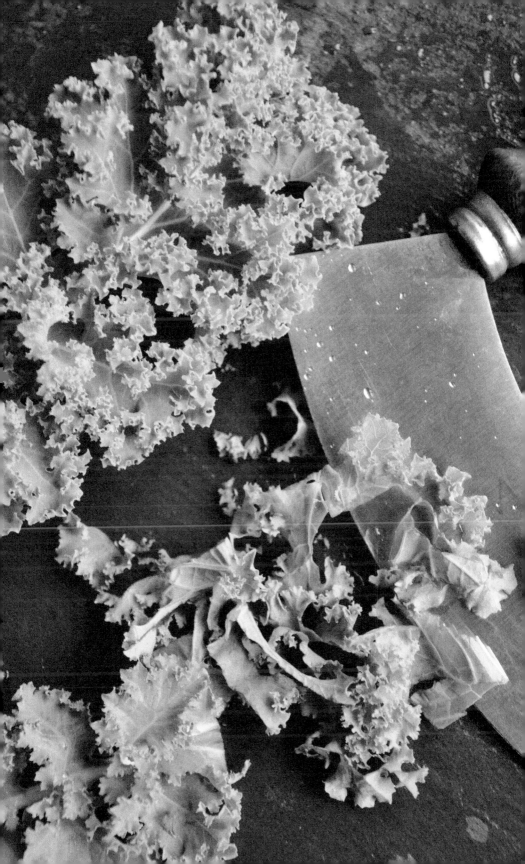

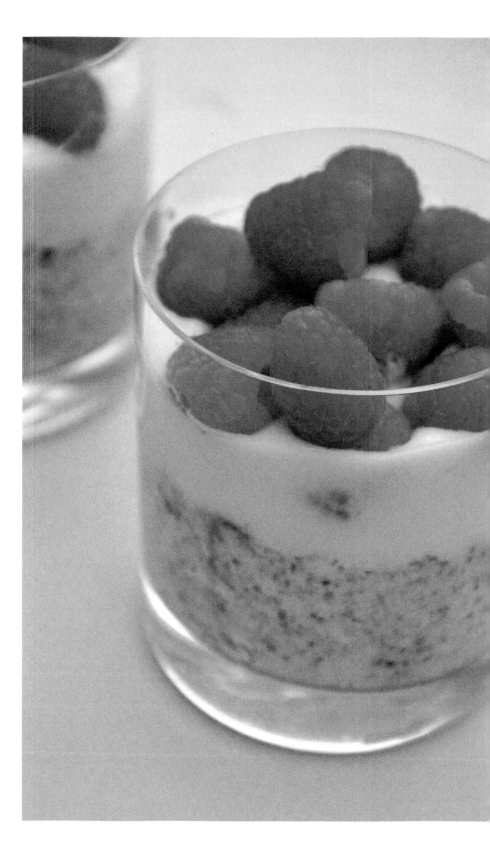

FLAX MUESLI WITH KUZU COCONUT CREAM
(Serves 2)

INGREDIENTS
For the muesli:
¼ cup (25g) ground flax seeds
¹/³ cup (30g) chopped almonds or cashews
¼ cup (25g) grated coconut
¼ cup (35g) oat bran
¼ cup (30g) raisins
I tsp cinnamon

For the kuzu coconut cream:
200ml sugar-free coconut/almond milk
I tsp pure vanilla extract
2 tbsp kuzu
4 tbsp live natural yoghurt

METHOD
1. Soak the muesli ingredients overnight in just enough water to cover.
2. Heat the coconut/almond milk in a pan with the vanilla extract until warm but not boiling.
3. Dissolve the kuzu in a little cold water to make a smooth paste and add to the warm milk.
4. Heat through, stirring constantly. Simmer for 3–5 minutes until the mixture thickens.
5. Let it cool and thicken, then mix with the yoghurt and pour on the muesli.
6. Serve with berries or fresh fruit of your choice

SWEDE & CAULIFLOWER MASH WITH FRESH SAGE & ROSEMARY
(Serves 2–3)

INGREDIENTS
Cauliflower head cut into florets
Swede peeled and cut into chunks
½ tsp salt ½ cup (60g) ground flaxseeds
2 tbsp coconut butter
2 tsp gomasio (sesame seed seasoning available from health shops)
½ tsp turmeric
I tsp dried sage or finely chopped fresh sage leaves

METHOD
1. Cook the cauliflower and swede together in a large pan of salty water until soft (the salt in the water stops the nutrients leaching out)
2. Drain and place in a large bowl
3. Mash and mix with the remaining ingredient
4. Let it stand for 5 minutes or until it sets into the desired consistency

MOOD AND BRAIN BOOSTING RECIPES

TRYPTOPHAN
Foods rich in tryptophan include game and turkey meat, spirulina, spinach and sesame seeds. Tryptophan is a precursor to serotonin, an important neurotransmitter involved in mood regulation and targeted by common antidepressants.

MUCUNA SEEDS
Contain significant levels of serotonin, tryptophan and L-dopa (a dopamine precursor) which boost brain dopamine and serotonin levels. Mucuna is potent and should be limited to 1tsp of powder per day unless under the supervision of a qualified practitioner.

OILY FISH
Omega-3s are components of brain tissue and protect the brain, improve memory and maintain neurological health and wellbeing.

CACAO & VERY DARK CHOCOLATE (70% COCOA)
Cacao refers to the raw, fermented, de-fatted, ground cocoa beans. Cocoa is similar but has also been roasted. The mood-boosting virtues of chocolate are attributed to a number of compounds ranging from resveratrol, an antioxidant and immune system booster which stimulates endorphins (natural opiates) and serotonin in the brain, to phenylethylamine (PEA) and anandamide. PEA is an adrenal-related chemical produced naturally when we're excited or fall in love, and anandamide resembles a chemical found in marijuana (THC) that binds to the endocannabinoid receptors in the brain. The endocannabinoid system is involved in the control of mood and anxiety –and a variety of neurological and cell-regulating functions.

CHILI AND CAYENNE PEPPER
Chilli peppers contain capsaicinoids which give them their heat. By tricking the brain into thinking that we are being burnt capsaicinoids activate the release of endorphins known to relieve pain and induce euphoria. The effect of endorphin release can last for up to an hour.

LIVER
The richest food in vitamin B12 and other key B vitamins necessary for energy production and nervous system health.

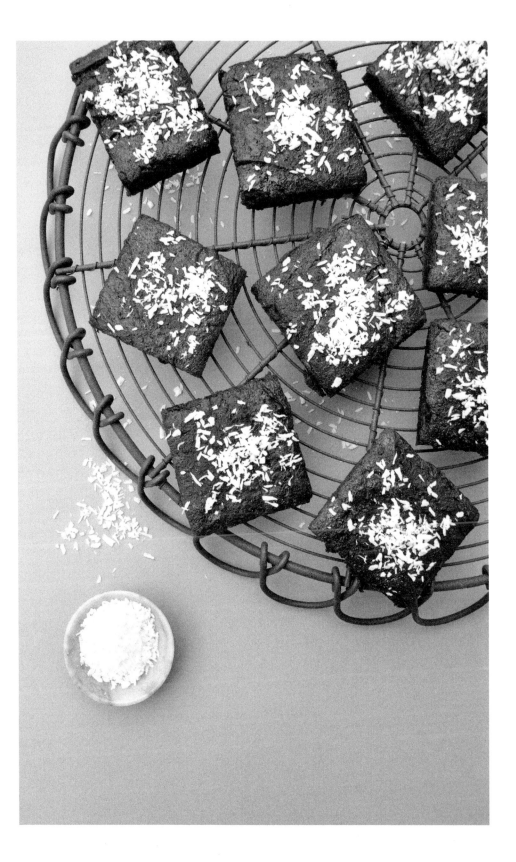

CHICKEN LIVER, FENNEL & SPINACH
(Serves 4)

INGREDIENTS

125g spinach, rinsed
and chopped
2 tbsp butter
1 fennel bulb, trimmed,
quartered and sliced,
(reserve a few fronds
for garnish)
2 garlic cloves, minced
225g chicken livers,
trimmed and sliced
100ml chicken stock or
port
4 anchovy fillets, rinsed
and chopped
1 tbsp capers, chopped
1 tsp dried sage
Salt and pepper, to
season

METHOD

1. Divide the spinach between 4 salad plates.
2. In a large frying pan, melt 1 tablespoon of the butter over a medium heat; add fennel and cook for about 3 minutes or until tender. Remove from frying pan and set aside.
3. In the pan, heat the remaining butter, add the garlic and cook for 1 minute.
4. Add the chicken livers and cook for 3–4 minutes or until no longer pink in the centre.
5. Return the fennel to the pan. Add the stock (or port), anchovies, capers, sage, salt and pepper and ook over a high heat for 2–3 minutes or until sauce is reduced slightly.
6. Spoon the mixture over individual salads and garnish with fennel fronds. Serve immediately

CHOCOLATE AND MUCUNA BROWNIES
(Makes 10 brownies)

INGREDIENTS

1 cup (100g) ground almonds

2 tbsp (15g) mucuna (also called velvet bean) powder*

1 tsp baking soda

2 medium to large sweet potatoes

15 Medjool dates (fleshier and softer than ordinary dates) stone removed

3 eggs

8 tbsp raw cacao (a good quality pure or organic cocoa)

4 tbsp coconut butter

Pinch salt

Pinch cayenne pepper (optional)

METHOD

1. Soak the dates for a few hours in 100ml of water.

2. Pre-heat oven to 320F/160°C/fan oven 140°C/ gas mark 3.

3. Peel, chop and cook the sweet potatoes in a steamer until they are very soft.

4. In a bowl thoroughly mix the ground almonds, mucuna powder and baking soda.

5. Place the dates with their water in a blender and blend until smooth

6. Add the cooked sweet potato chunks, cacao, eggs, salt, cayenne pepper (if using) and coconut butter

7. Continue to blend until smooth and creamy.

8. Tip into a bowl and mix with the dried ingredients.

9. Place into a lined baking shallow dish and cook for about 40 minutes. Pierce with a knife to check that it is cooked through. When it comes out clean, it's ready.

10. Remove from the tray and allow to cool for at least 10 minutes before cutting into squares.

*Available to order from Indigo Herbs http://www.indigo-herbs.co.uk/

Index

ACKNOWLEDGEMENTS

I would like to thank my parents and teachers for teaching me to ask questions and for nourishing my passion for life, health and biology.

I must also express my profound gratitude to: Francine Lawrence for her tireless and meticulous support in the creation of this book, without her it would still be a dream; Brian Miller for his encouragement and for his contribution to the ideas I have developed in this book; and Nicola Yuen for her clear page layouts and creative cover design.

Finally, I would like to thank my many supportive friends who have all participated in this project in different ways — and everyone who has consulted me and taught me something about the miracle of life.

ANNE-LISE MILLER
HEALTH-STYLE FOR LIFE

Anne-Lise Miller, Therapist & Author

If you have found this book useful and would like to know more about nutrition and Anne-Lise's systemic approach to health, please visit her website (details below). You will find nutritional information, news about latest research, articles about health, advice on detoxing, plus delicious sugar- and gluten-free recipes. You can also sign up for Anne-Lise's quarterly newsletter to receive the latest news about her projects and programmes, including her Detox Retreats.

Anne-Lise Miller is based in London and works from her practice in Hampstead. She has a scientific background and studied biology, and has been a naturopathic practitioner for over 25 years. One of the leading teachers of colonic hydrotherapy in the UK, Anne-Lise is an internationally renowned expert on the subject, and holds qualifications in colonic hydrotherapy, aromatherapy, massage, kinesiology, nutritional counselling, exercise, hypnotherapy and psychotherapy.

Anne-Lise Miller Detox Retreats in France

A detox retreat is not only a wonderful way to shape up and get your health back after over-indulging; it is a unique opportunity to clear your thinking and release yourself from the habitual chatter of the mind. Letting go of the toxic mental and physical burdens that limit health and vitality frequently helps to resolve issues creatively; it will also show you how to find new solutions and establish healthier choices once you are back home.

Join a small group of like-minded people for a week of juices, counselling, yoga, massage and regular colonic treatments led by Anne-Lise herself, in the clear mountain air of the Pyrenees. Lift the brain fog, wake up your system and relax in a peaceful space. After a week of detoxing you will return feeling healthier and more relaxed. Dates for the next Detox Retreats can be found on the website.

If you would like to buy more copies of this book to give to your friends, and for more information and recipes, please visit: www.annelisemiller.com

Lightning Source UK Ltd.
Milton Keynes UK
UKOW07f1645280816

281638UK00008B/45/P